EBURY PRESS

SACRED

Vasudha Rai is a bestselling author, columnist, podcaster and an award-winning journalist who has written on beauty and wellness for more than two decades. Her first book, *Glow: Indian Foods, Recipes and Rituals for Beauty, Inside & Out*, revived the usage of traditional ingredients in everyday living. Her second book, *Ritual: Daily Practices for Wellness, Beauty & Bliss*, modernizes traditional practices for contemporary lifestyles. A yoga teacher with a 300-hour certification, Vasudha has taught yoga at The Yoga Studio in Delhi.

Her beauty columns have appeared in *The Hindu Weekend* and *HT Mint Lounge*. Two seasons of her podcast 'Holistic Healing with Vasudha Rai'—in association with RedFM, India's leading radio channel—are streaming across all major platforms, including Spotify, Jio Saavn, Google Podcasts and Apple Podcasts. Her work has appeared in publications such as *Vogue*, *Condé Nast Traveller* and *The Hindu Weekend*. In the past, she has been the beauty director for *Harper's Bazaar*, *Cosmopolitan* and *Women's Health India*.

In 2019, Vasudha was awarded the Beauty & Wellness Voice of the Year at the *Cosmopolitan* Blogger Awards. In 2022, she was awarded the Voice of Reason in Beauty Writing as part of the *Vogue* Beauty Festival, and the Future Forward Influencer in the Wellness category by *Peaklife* magazine. In 2024, Vasudha released her audiobook, an Audible Original titled 'The Book of Holistic Beauty'. These days, Vasudha enjoys writing books, interacting with her Instagram audience and gardening at her home in Gurugram, India.

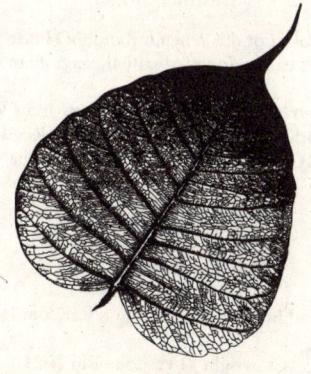

SACRED

The MYSTICISM, SCIENCE, RECIPES & RITUALS

around the plants we worship

VASUDHA RAI

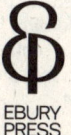

EBURY
PRESS

An imprint of Penguin Random House

EBURY PRESS

Ebury Press is an imprint of the Penguin Random House group of companies
whose addresses can be found at global.penguinrandomhouse.com

Published by Penguin Random House India Pvt. Ltd
4th Floor, Capital Tower 1, MG Road,
Gurugram 122 002, Haryana, India

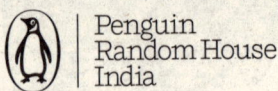

First published in Ebury Press by Penguin Random House India 2025

Copyright © Vasudha Rai 2025

Illustrations by Akangksha Sarmah

ISBN 9780143469353

Typeset in Adobe Garamond Pro by Manipal Technologies Limited, Manipal
Printed at Thomson Press India Ltd, New Delhi

www.penguin.co.in

For Krishna and Rishaan, the divine gifts in my life.
And my parents, my soulmates.

CONTENTS

CONTENTS

PART III: SANCTIFY

FOREWORD

There was a time when humans used to live over large swathes of land, sit under a wide canopy of trees, bathe in rivers and walk in lush green forests. But over the last couple of decades, our lives have shrunk and become nano-sized. Today, we are limited to our smartphones and tiny apartments. I call them cellular heavens, which don't go beyond the virtual world and are limited to four walls, be it in cafes, malls or hotels. As we shrink, we lose sight of the bigger picture, the biodiversity and the rhythms of nature. And as technology leapfrogs every week, leading to the need to adapt quickly, we don't have the patience to plant something and watch it grow.

There is a culture of swiping through things, which permeates into our relationships, friendships and businesses. Because of this, it seems as if nothing is stable. Our attention spans have shortened and that is affecting all our activities, especially our commitment towards nature, which still moves at its own pace. Alarmingly though, the pace of extinction of plant and animal species has sped up because of massive deforestation. While this happens, we are distracted by the daily worries of job security and traffic. But the biggest distraction is climate change, a concern we assume is lurking decades into the future, so we ignore the small steps that will provide long-term respite, such as the planting of trees and preservation of forests.

Today, humans live in an unconscious state, without any pauses, contemplation, discussion or signs of slowing down. Therefore, we are far removed from awareness of our destructive actions, which are catapulting our descent into a catastrophic future. If the recent spike in pollution is something to go by, we must be very alarmed and act quickly, or, at the very least, preserve whatever is left of our natural resources.

Though we view plants and water bodies as sacred, we don't care for them because we assume that divinity will take care of itself. In addition, plants and trees are being plundered during religious months; for instance, bael trees being torn apart during Shivaratri or banyan trees during folk rituals. There is no real connection, it seems as if we are just fulfilling a formality for personal gain. Our worship is transactional—if I tie a thread around a tree or offer leaves to god, I will be blessed with abundance. But true worship is when we respect nature and work towards its protection. Because when we preserve and care for our natural resources, the rewards—clean air, biodiversity and enriched soil—are priceless.

If you pause and think about how perfectly balanced natural processes are, you cannot help but be astounded at this miraculous and wonderful world. Chlorophyll is god and oxygen is a divine blessing. It's mind blowing that oceans produce 50 per cent of oxygen, which comes from plankton and algae. The most obvious benefit of planting, preserving and growing trees is that it provides shade, which helps reduce temperatures and thereby control global warming. More trees mean an increase in biodiversity, more insect population, and more microbes and more lichens, which occupy almost 7 per cent of the Earth's land surface. Without lichens, there will be no soil in the forests. They grow on trees and have their own intelligence that produces over 20,000 species of itself in the world. Lichens are just one example of the wonders of the natural world. I consider nature to be miraculous. Because of this, for me, there are four Vedas: air, water, soil and forests. Air, water and soil are created by forests.

In the past year, there has been a growing interest in sustainability from a marketing point of view. But not everything can be monetized because some things are priceless: love, time, happiness, companionship and the preservation of natural resources. The natural world works relentlessly for us and does not understand the language of money. Today, we are creating a world that is dominated by artificial intelligence (AI), but we have forgotten about 1.3 billion-year-old plant intelligence, or PI—without it, there is no us. We've only been around for 2,00,000 years, but plants have been creating and sculpting the earth and giving birth to various species for several millennia. Never forget that we are birthed from this PI and not from AI, which is enslaving us rapidly. All religions say that there is an overriding intelligence, and by that they refer to this rhythm and intelligence of nature. Though we follow our religions, we have forgotten how to respect nature—the purest form of worship. Among humans, it's only the indigenous tribes who still understand this and respect ancestral and plant intelligence.

If we continue to plunder and destroy natural resources, do you think nature will sit back and do nothing? It has been proved through millions of years that nature does not allow a single species to dominate: be it dinosaurs, mammoths or sabre-toothed tigers. What makes you think that it will allow humans to rule the planet while they plunder the earth? Though we may have dominated for several millennia, if we are not relevant to the health of this planet, we will be eliminated. Never forget that nature is beneficial to humans, and not the other way around. It is estimated that every day more than a hundred species go extinct. What makes you think we won't be next?

Swami Prem Parivartan, fondly known as 'Peepal Baba', environmentalist and founder of the Give Me Trees Trust, which has planted over 25 million trees

INTRODUCTION

It is a few days past Navaratri, a festival where the goddess is worshipped for nine days in a row. Now that the celebrations are over and we have officially entered the auspicious time of the year, a few people are gathered near my house to axe an ancient tree, which (barely grazing their plot) needs to be removed to make way for stilt parking. The irony doesn't escape my notice: On the one hand, we worship the various forms of the goddess and on the other, we plunder the earth, which is the most relevant goddess for us humans. Our planet provides us food and shelter. The trees that nourish the earth goddess provide us with precious oxygen, enrich the soil and prevent its erosion. Trees also provide shade and opportunities for economic growth, whether it is through farming, enriching the soil or providing shelter. But since humans lack foresight, we slaughter forests to make way for human settlements and only focus on short-term gains. We forget that nurturing nature means nurturing ourselves and everything man-made increases toxicity and pollution.

It's a common misconception we see not just in India but all over the world where trees are being hacked in the name of development to make way for roads, statues and buildings. Recent research has shown that deforestation is a global catastrophe, with almost 16 million acres razed just in 2023, despite 140 countries pledging to halt deforestation. What does that have to do with us you ask? The most direct impact of deforestation is a rise in the number of diseases, for instance, malaria, dengue, Ebola and SARS. These microbes were limited to forests and living in harmony with the animals and birds who had adapted to these bacteria and viruses. But as we lose forests, we are coming in closer contact with animals who host these microbes, increasing the frequency and severity of infections. SARS, Covid-19, Ebola, are just a few examples of such diseases. Additionally, since trees help prevent soil erosion, a decrease in their numbers means soil depletion, reduced agricultural productivity and an increase in the occurrence of catastrophes, such as flooding and landslides. Not to mention the daily loss of hundreds of plant and animal species, all due to rapid deforestation, which leads to a change in climate and the environment.

The problem begins when we consider ourselves to be the primary inhabitants of this planet and view trees as inanimate, instead of respecting them as divine beings like we did in earlier centuries. There was a time when man worshipped the elements of nature that sustained humankind. We showed great reverence and respect for trees, rivers, sunlight and other natural resources. But worship today has reached such a crescendo that we are devoted to an intangible god but do not respect tangible manifestations of the divine, such as plants, soil and water bodies. In certain religions around the world, trees are revered as gods and branches are seen as the universe. Some trees and plants are believed to have originated from parts of the bodies and limbs of gods; for instance, the rudraksha tree is believed to have originated from the tears of Lord Shiva. Then there are plants that are considered to be a bridge between us and the supernatural world and medicinal plants that are believed to be the abode of gods and nature spirits.

In the *shastras*, or holy scriptures, it is said that one who plants one each of peepal, neem and banyan; ten tamarind, three each of wood apple, holy bael and myrobalan, and five mango trees goes to heaven. Superstitious as it may be, if every human were to plant all these trees and ensured that they grew to full maturity, we would have several billion more trees. Therefore, divine botany, which is the study of the relationship between plants and humans based on faith and tradition, must be explored and revived.

In this time of climate change, as we accelerate towards catastrophe, we often hear people say that humans are destroying the planet, which reflects the enormity of the human ego. How can we assume ourselves to be so powerful that we destroy a planet that has withstood the test of time and has seen several species inhabit its land over millions of years? The truth is that we aren't just destroying the planet; we are eliminating life as we know it. By plundering natural resources, we are in the process of making the earth completely inhabitable for us but are also annihilating the chances of our survival. So, who are we to destroy the planet? We are only destroying ourselves.

This book hopes to serve as a reminder that we should live in harmony with nature and that plants around us are a form of divinity and should be treated as such. According to ancient scriptures, every leaf and blade of grass, branch and the trunk of every tree is home to nature spirits. There is an ancient tale in which a guru asks his disciple to go into the forest and find a plant that has no use. The disciple comes back empty-handed because he couldn't find a single plant that had no use. This is why every plant must be seen as sacred because every species supports some sort of bacteria, insects, birds, bees, butterflies and mammals, which has concomitant benefits for the entire planet and humanity. Some plants enrich the soil with their mere presence, while others purify the air. There are also those that preserve the groundwater table and prevent flooding.

As temperatures grow warmer and seasons more severe, the biggest benefit of plants is their ability to keep the surroundings cool. Despite the fact that summer is getting hotter and the monsoon more catastrophic, trees that populated our forests, mountains and riverbanks are cut down to make way for so-called development. Can we really consider this progress when it leads to an increase in temperature, depletes water tables and diminishes air quality? Perhaps the solution lies in us looking at plants as divine creatures. True worship is, however, not limited to offering *prasad* to a tree or lighting a diya for prayer. It is about showing our reverence by preserving forests and green cover, which nourish us, our water tables, the soil and air quality. Plants absorb about 30 per cent of carbon dioxide in the air each year. They also help improve soil quality and reduce extreme temperature fluctuations. Forests retain excess rainwater and prevent floods. By holding this excess water in the soil, they help return it to the atmosphere. Trees also help keep the water bodies clean, as they intercept and trap sediments instead of them flowing directly into streams and rivers.

Where there are trees, there is shade. Therefore, planting trees and preventing them from being cut is a better strategy to mitigate climate change, than say, drinking through a paper straw. Ultimately, it is not cement and concrete that will protect and nourish us from the assaults of the environment. It is trees and plants that help nourish the ecosystem from the ground up. It is the green cover that provides us valuable oxygen and shade to keep temperatures cool. Without vegetation, there will be no humankind. By vegetation I don't mean the over-fertilized monocultures of agriculture today, but biodiverse landscapes with trees, herbs, grains and fruits grown together to enrich the land and provide better sources of income to the farmers.

The problem is that we just expect change to happen, whereas true change begins with the recognition that there is indeed a problem, and small steps are taken to resolve it. For instance, plant a tree on your birthday as a minimum. But more importantly, prevent fully grown trees from being cut, as they are an ecosystem in themselves. A fully grown tree can never be replaced with a new sapling. Because how can you replace something that has taken twenty to fifty years to fully mature? How can we replace an ancient tree that has deep roots and a wide canopy that is now home to thousands of species of microbes, birds, butterflies, insects and other small animals, not to mention the oxygen and shade that a fully grown tree provides us? This intrinsic value of nature and trees was understood by tribals all over the world who still respect nature and worship sacred forests even to this day. In India, we have scriptures dedicated to the divine presence in various plants. But surprisingly, very few large-scale studies have been conducted so far to discern the benefits of these sacred plants. To appreciate the immense value of green cover, one has to be interested in plants. What is the scientific basis of these beliefs? What are the medicinal benefits? Why are some trees associated with gods? How do different species of trees intersect among various faiths? The material is all there, but we need more studies to develop divine botany as a robust science, which will, in turn, spur conservation efforts. This book hopes to get this conversation started.

If we delve deep into the science of divine botany, we observe that humans connected with plants on three broad parameters: first, as a vehicle for connection with the divine; second, as an offering during prayer; and third, to purify homes and places of worship. Keeping these three parameters in mind, this book has been divided into three sections:

1. SEEK

These are the plants we utilize to find a connection with the universe. Whether it is burning guggul or frankincense to send prayers to the universe via their cloudy, fragrant smoke; consuming cannabis or dhatura to be in a state of hypnosis that opens up a portal to the divine; or simply detoxifying the body with a fruit such as haritaki to prepare for meditation. The plants suggested in this part of the book are chosen by seekers as a link with divine energy.

2. SURRENDER

The path towards worship always begins by seeking but settles into surrender, a state of mind where we are truly open to the acts of god. In this part of the book, I have listed the plants, fruits and flowers that are offered to the divine or utilized in purification rituals. This includes the aphrodisiac effect of a paan leaf as well as the purifying effect of a miswak twig on the teeth. It also includes fruits such as pomegranate and jujube, as well as fragrant flowers such as jasmine and parijat, which are offered to gods and goddesses.

3. SANCTIFY

Ever since the beginning of civilization, plants have often been used to sanctify spaces. In ancient Greek and Roman times, it was the fig and olive tree; in ancient Egypt, it was trees such as frankincense and myrrh, and in India, there are plants such as tulsi, among many others, which were believed to enhance the energy and purity of the area around them. While there are many superstitions associated with such plants, this book hopes to demystify the folklore surrounding some of these plants and why they are worthy of worship.

The chapters cover several rituals, recipes and benefits related to these plants. However, it is essential to realize that plants, shrubs, trees, creepers, etc., benefit us even by their mere presence. There are several studies today to prove that time spent with nature benefits humans physically, mentally and emotionally. And as the world gets urbanized at a rapid pace, this book hopes to give you pause and understand that true growth is when we grow in harmony with nature. When we destroy natural resources, we are only eliminating our health and happiness. With this book, my endeavour is to provide you with foresight and to make you fall in love with plants, which have always served us well.

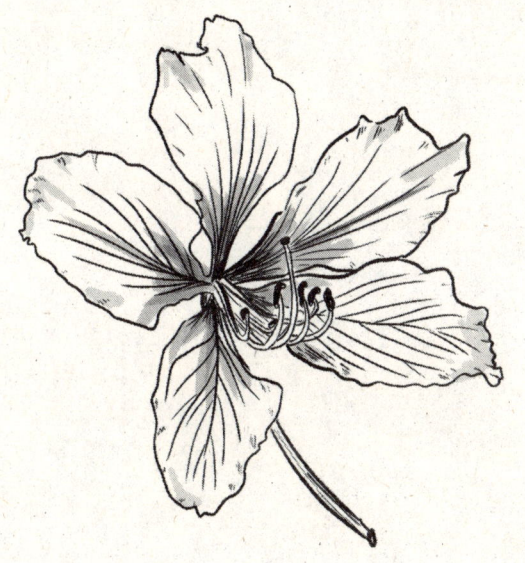

PART I

Seek

INTRODUCTION

Who is a seeker? Are they people who accept the concept of spirituality as it is or do they start their own inquiry to find their version of spiritual truth? Whether you are seeking god, a connection with the universe or a peek into your own consciousness, these are all different versions of the same journey. It begins with a desire to look beyond the daily routine, to find something more sublime than what we perceive with our senses. The idea of a divine presence is manifested in many ways. Some look for it in idols, others find it in stillness, many find it in action and charity, while there are some for whom divinity is woven into everyday life—it is a part of their every breath, every action and every word.

Typically, the divine is seen as something greater than us, something that nourishes and protects us. Perhaps that is why in the ancient times, man worshipped plants and trees, rivers, the sun and the moon. These elements helped nourish our bodies, gave us shelter, and the stars and the moon even gave ancient travellers direction. In the past, there was the awareness that we are just a microcosm of the macrocosm. Man knew that there were things greater than us, for instance plants, which are essential for our survival and were seen as having their own unique spirit. Over the years, as man became the most powerful creature on the planet, he brushed aside the relevance and sanctity of natural resources and started to have unshakeable faith in his own creations, which we now know come with their own downsides. Every man-made advancement only provided temporary relief, as their accompanying side effects were responsible for long-term destruction. But on the other hand, when we turn back to nature's rhythms, it is often less expensive, more beneficial and without any unseen side effects.

Indeed, connecting with nature is the first step to seek the divine. While traditionally, shamans and sadhus utilized plants to reach a state of hypnosis, it remains an advanced practice. For me, simply sitting under a tree or watering a plant is a direct connection with the universe. These everyday rituals have been proven to help us achieve a state of calmness and to reduce anxiety. One must never forget that plants were the original inhabitants of this planet and the first creation of divine force. It's no surprise then that spending time with plants—whether by indulging in a nature walk or gardening—significantly reduces stress levels. Even just looking at plants has been found to reduce stress, fear, anger and sadness, as well as alleviate blood pressure, pulse rate and muscle tension. Another study of post-operative patients found that just observing certain species of indoor plants helps reduce the severity of one's pain and duration of stay in a hospital. Therefore, every spiritual journey begins by interacting with nature. If you seek the divine, then begin with the worship of nature.

In Part I, I have outlined the herbs, resins, flowers and fruits that refine the consciousness and help us begin our journey as a seeker. Whether it's through a fragrant resin or a detoxifying fruit, there are many ways to begin walking the path, and it starts here, in the embrace of sacred nature.

FRANKINCENSE AND MYRRH

The common thread running through most
cultures of the world is the use of fragrance
in religious ceremonies. Why is it that we
use perfumes when we seek the divine?
Some believe that certain scents purify
and cleanse a space, making it worthy of
angelic and divine presence. Others use
it as a part of their daily prayer and many
consider fragrance as an etheric vehicle to
carry prayers to the universe.

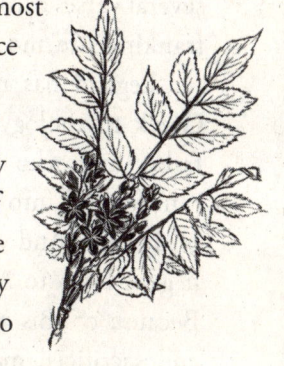

Among all divine scents, frankincense and myrrh are
known as holy smoke since they are regularly used to
consecrate and sanctify places of worship. Their most
popular association is that they were two of the three gifts
of Magi—the first gift being gold—which the three wise
men gifted to baby Jesus. Symbolically, gold represents
the kingly aspect of Christ, frankincense his divine
side and myrrh, which was commonly used to
embalm bodies, foretold his tragic yet graceful
death. Pliny the Elder, the Roman scholar who
authored the encyclopaedic *Natural History*,
wrote that members of the families who retained
the hereditary right of trading in frankincense

were deemed sacred and were therefore not allowed to be polluted by salacious activities or a funeral procession during the process of obtaining resin from the trees. It is rumoured that the Roman emperor Nero burned a year's production of frankincense at the funeral of his wife, Poppaea. The Chinese called frankincense 'fanhunxiang', meaning 'calling back the dead fragrance'. In the Bible, several verses extoll the sensorial effect of spices, particularly frankincense and myrrh.

Legend has it that Myrrha, the mother of Adonis in Greek mythology, who had an incestuous passion for her father and who tricked him into sleeping with her, was transformed into a myrrh tree and her tears became the sap of the tree. And when the myrrh tree was split by an arrow, it gave birth to Adonis, the child of a father and daughter. Because of this association, myrrh is used both in sensual and sacrificial manner, either in fragrance or at sacrificial altars. Myrrh was also offered to Isis, the Egyptian goddess of death and mourning. Contrastingly, the Romans drank wine flavoured with different herbs and spices, including myrrh. In fact, Pliny the Elder also states that tree resins were used to remove unwanted hair from men's bodies.

In ancient times, the production of these resins was limited to the Horn of Africa and the kingdom of Sheba (presently Yemen and Ethiopia). Pliny wrote that since these resins were prized for their use in worship and perfumery, this trade made the Arabs the richest race on earth. They had a monopoly over the limited areas where these resins grew wild and they also kept a tight lease on the routes their caravans used in bringing these products. Keep in mind that these resins were more expensive than gold. Therefore, the region where these trees grew wild (i.e., Yemen and its surrounding areas) came to be known as Arabia Felix, meaning 'Blessed Arabia' or 'Fortunate Arabia'. Think of it like this: Out of the 100 million sesterces (ancient Roman coins) spent on importing resins from the East, more than half were spent on incense from Arabia.

The word 'perfume' is derived from the Latin phrase 'per fumum', which means 'by smoke', whereas 'incense' is derived from the Latin word 'incendere', meaning that which is lit. Frankincense was first known as olibanum, a term that was probably derived from the Arabic 'al laben' or 'al luban' meaning 'white', as the white tears of this resins are the most valuable. Even in Hebrew, it is known as levona, which also means white and colloquially in India, we call it loban. The Egyptian word for myrrh was 'bal', which meant 'sweeping out', signifying its medicinal and spiritual properties. Queen Hatshepsut was so enamoured by these trees that she had them uprooted from the Land of Punt (probably modern-day Somalia, which still exports these precious resins) and had them planted in Egypt. These trees are depicted as part of Egyptian hieroglyphics and even a stump of Hatshepsut's myrrh tree is present in Luxor, at her mortuary on the banks of the Nile.

The Science

Scents are deeply intertwined with mood and memory. Our positive and negative associations with fragrance can differ according to the ingredient used and, more importantly, the memory related to that particular fragrance. Our sense of smell is controlled by neurons within tissue placed high inside the nasal cavity and connect directly to the brain. What we perceive as flavour is strongly connected to our olfactory abilities. Additionally, the olfactory bulb located in the front of our brain sends signals to the limbic system, including the amygdala, which detects danger, and the hippocampus, which works on memory and emotions. This is why scents hold so much power over memory; you may forget an incident, but one whiff of a particular smell and it all comes rushing back.

In 2008, a small animal study showed that a chemical found in frankincense may elevate mood. *Incensole acetate*, a component of the Boswellia plant, was injected in mice and it was found that this worked as a mild drug that was about ten times less potent than valium in the reduction of anxiety. One of the parameters of the anxiety test was a fear of open spaces: injected mice were found to be less fearful than those who weren't. Studies have also found that both frankincense and myrrh essential oils and fumes show reduction in airborne microbes. To be more specific, 45.39 per cent reduction of airborne fungi and 67.56 per cent reduction for bacteria with the smoke of these resins when they were fumigated. And 80.43 per cent reduction for fungi and 91.43 per cent for bacteria when the essential oil of these resins was burned. It has also been found that the use of Casperome, a purified mixture of triterpenoid extracts from frankincense, may be beneficial for asthma patients, as it helps reduce the frequency of inhalation therapy. But of course, asthmatic patients must check with their pulmonologist before trying any holistic remedies.

Frankincense extract also helps enhance memory in elderly patients. Additionally, the inhalation of its essential oil showed positive effects on the reduction of labour pains. Frankincense is a wonderful addition to skincare too, as it has demonstrated wound-healing properties by inducing wound contraction. Because of these healing qualities, it has also shown promise in healing peptic and colon ulcers.

Myrrh is used as a mouthwash, primarily for its antiseptic properties—the same quality that made it popular in the ancient world as an embalming agent. In Traditional Chinese Medicine (TCM), myrrh, also known as 'mo yao', is used to treat amenorrhoea, abdominal pain, injuries and broken bones. Interestingly, in Ayurveda, where it is known as guggul, it is used for the same purposes. In fact, in the seventh century, there was a balsam made by a priest in a Franciscan Monastery of Jerusalem (which was known for its outstanding apothecary). This balsam, made with frankincense, myrrh, aloe and mastic, was revered in Europe and the Near East for its antiseptic, anti-inflammatory and antioxidant properties. Though it lost its popularity by the late nineteenth century, it's a reminder of how these sacred ingredients were interwoven into the fabric of daily life.

The fact is that both these resins contain potent anti-inflammatory compounds. When inflammation happens (due to injuries, infections or disorders of the immune system), the body produces leukotrienes, which are small mediator chemicals that promote free radicals, autoimmune responses and other processes that trigger inflammation. Another study compared the effect of myrrh to that of Prednisolone in the treatment of autoimmune diseases. In the two groups of mice, the ones injected with myrrh extract showed a slight decrease in inflammatory cell count as compared to the group injected with Prednisolone, where there was a marked decrease. Nevertheless, myrrh did help reduce the side effect of Prednisolone in the liver, which shows that it can possibly be beneficial as a conjunctive therapy in combination with mainstream medicine.

Application

Resins are part of the Torchwood family (Burseraceae), or simply put, the incense family of trees. These trees themselves are nothing spectacular to look at, but if you think about the harsh environment they grow in, you'll have nothing but respect for these hardy trees. The roots, which grow into barren cliffs and boulders made of limestone, are good at absorbing water. Therefore, even if there is barely any rainfall in these regions, the trees thrive by tapping into small reserves of water from the limestone. Myrrh is a thorny shrub or tree that can grow up to 12 feet in height, even in hot, sunny and dry conditions. As both trees are native to arid climates, it's hard to grow them everywhere.

Even if you cannot grow them in your garden, these resins can be made a part of your routine to elevate everyday living. You can toss organic myrrh and frankincense resins into rosewater to infuse it with their benefits. Or use them to purify the environment at home. I personally love burning these resins to clear the energy of my home.

How to Burn Regrant Resins

Ingredients

A charcoal puck/ a charcoal cup/ or a cow dung *havan* cup
½ tsp of a single or mixed resins

Method

If you're using a puck or a tablet, opt for a pair of tongs to hold them over a candle so that it burns evenly. When it has burnt around the edges, place it in a resin burner or atop a metal diya and sprinkle the frankincense and myrrh resins on top. Make sure you don't place the charcoal table on a glass bowl or plate, which has the tendency to crack because of the heat.

If you are using a charcoal or cow dung havan cup, just light the rim till it releases smoke and fill in the resins. Sometimes I like to hold the cup with a pair of tongs over a lit gas stove. Use a resin burner or metal diya to place the cup. Sometimes we cannot burn frankincense and myrrh resins because they may cause pollution or someone in the family has asthma. In such cases, it's better to burn essential oils of these resins. For this, you need to add a sprinkle of water to an oil burner. To this, add a few drops of these oils and light a beeswax candle underneath to heat and disperse the oil.

Of course, the shortcut method of using essential oils is to dab them on lightbulbs and then switch them on. The heat from the bulbs helps activate and disperse the oils.

Purification Ritual with Frankincense

Ingredients

Frankincense resin
Myrrh resin
Water (use Gangajal or any holy water)
A small amount of alcohol (as a preservative)

Instructions

- Grind the frankincense and myrrh resins to make a fine powder. Take equal amounts of myrrh and frankincense. Now add a small amount of alcohol (vodka works well because it's odourless) to the powder.
- Boil 300 ml water for two–three minutes, and then let it cool slightly.
- Add the powdered resins to the warm water and mix it anticlockwise.
- Allow the mixture to sit for at least twenty-four hours; the longer it infuses, the stronger the potion will be. Putting the mixture under moonlight, preferably in waning moon, will energize the mixture.
- Energize with incantations: You may chant the following nine times:

Under the waning moon's gentle decline,
I call on your power, oh moon, intertwine.

As you wane, so too shall the energies we abhor,
Remove negativity, open the purification door.
Frankincense and myrrh, resins so old,
Infuse this potion with powers bold.
Guardians of the sacred, keepers of the night,
Bless this brew with your celestial light.
Moon above, your cycle imparts,
A rhythm that calms and purifies hearts.
As you shrink, take away the taint,
Leave purity where there was complaint.
Let this mixture soak up thine essence rare,
Under starlit sky and cool night air.
Each passing night, as you disappear,
Fill this potion with power clear.
This brew I craft under the moon's watchful eyes,
To cleanse, to clear, to purify.
By the time the moon hides her face,
Let this potion be imbued with grace.

- Strain and bottle: Strain the mixture through a fine mesh or cheesecloth into a clean spray bottle. Use this spray to smudge the areas where burning resins isn't possible to cleanse and purify spaces of negative energies.

Meditation Bliss Blend

Ingredients

Frankincense (4 drops): Wonderfully grounding
Myrrh (3 drops): Has amazing depth and calming quality
Lavender (4 drops): Classic relaxation
Bergamot orange/Sweet orange (3 drops): Just a hint of uplifting energy
Jojoba oil (30 ml): Absorbs so well, you'll barely feel it

Method

Mix the essential oils together first. Add in the jojoba oil and shake well. Give it a little shake before each use. Apply 1–2 drops to your wrists, temples or behind your ears when you're ready to dive into meditation.

Note: Always do a little patch test first to make sure your skin's happy.

If you have sensitive skin or any allergies, maybe double-check with a healthcare professional. Keep your blends stored in a cool, dark spot so that they stay fresh.

HARITAKI

The story goes that when Indra, the Vedic god of rain and storms, was sipping *amrita,* or nectar, in heaven, a drop of this nectar fell on earth and through this sprouted the haritaki plant. Also known as *terminalia chebula*, it is considered to be the king of herbs in traditional medicine systems. So exalted is its status in Ayurveda, Tibetan medicine and TCM, that the iconography of Medicine Buddha shows him holding a begging bowl with the nectar of life in his right hand and the haritaki fruit or plant in his left hand. In Buddhism, it is considered to be the supreme nectar that illuminates the mind. In TCM, it is also known as the 'big golden fruit' because of its appearance, 'the wind floating fruit' for its ability to grow in harsh, arid conditions, while the Tibetans call it 'Arura', meaning that it is as valuable as a rhinoceros horn in terms of medicinal value.

Indian Buddhist monks introduced China not only to Buddhism but also to the benefits of this miraculous fruit. It is known as He Zi in Chinese, meaning 'speaking loudly and angrily', indicating the need for *haritaki*. In another tale, a girl named Yichaoma was gifted this tree by Medicine Buddha for her charity and helpfulness. The folklore is that Buddha told her that 'this is the best medicine in the world. Its roots, trunks and branches remove all diseases of the flesh, bone and skin, while its fruit can treat diseases of the internal organs'. In the Han Dynasty, an Indian monk visited the Guangxiao Temple and brought with him the haritaki plant.

The monks in the temple often chewed the fruits to quench their thirst as they chanted the sutras. Sometimes this fruit was decocted with licorice for pilgrims. In the Tang Dynasty, a decoction made from the three myrobalans (amla, baheda and haritaki—basically triphala) was immensely popular in the upper classes. In fact, when the famous poet Liu Yuxi fell severely ill with dysentery, he was given a pot of medicinal wine made from haritaki.

In Indian mythology, the tree is related to both Vishnu and Shiva, as Hari is another name for the preserver and Hara another name for the destroyer. The herb is mentioned in all Ayurvedic classics, nighantus and works on materia medica. Acharya Charaka, who is considered the father of Ayurveda, wrote that haritaki is the best among herbs that can be consumed regularly. Though Ayurvedic and Tibetan texts suggest seven different varieties of this fruit, the truth is that today only two varieties are used. There is the larger Vijaya variety, which is used for rejuvenation and purification. And there is the smaller variety (Jangi haritaki), which is the Chetaki variety, with stoneless fruits, approximately the breadth of a finger in size, used for medicinal and purgative purposes.

Though the haritaki fruit is primarily valued for its use in medicinal preparation, the whole tree is revered in Tibetan medicine. The roots are used to treat diseases of the bone, the stem for muscular diseases, the bark for skin, the branches for vascular disorders, the leaves for visceral organs, and the fruit for vital organs, including the heart. This humble tree, which requires barely anything to grow, offers us so much with every part of its being. It truly deserves its exalted, sacred status.

The Science

Haritaki today plays an important role, as it aids in detoxification and digestion. Ayurveda believes that the process of healing begins right at the taste buds. In this respect, haritaki contains five out of the six tastes in Ayurveda, i.e., sweet, sour, bitter, pungent and astringent. The only taste it doesn't have is salty. Because of the therapeutic effect of the combination of flavours, it is considered to be anti-inflammatory, anti-asthmatic, anti-pyretic, wound healing, good for rejuvenation and the best herb to clean the channels of the body. Its mild, purgative action helps control vata and this is also effective to reduce high levels of lipids, mainly cholesterol and triglycerides. This is why it is one of the three herbs in triphala considered to be a detoxifier and digestive.

A marked increase in both glutathione and superoxide dismutase (both potent antioxidants) have been found after treatment with haritaki extract. Several animal studies have shown that it helps reduce blood sugar, has shown promise in cardio-protective activity and has exhibited anti-fungal activity. However, the most applicable benefit of this herb is its purgative action. In Ayurveda, it is known as the anulomana effect, which means to break the bonds between faecal matter and intestinal mucosa for better elimination. And animal studies have found that haritaki churna (powder) significantly decreased the time it took to digest food in the intestine.

But that's not all. This wonderful herb has cosmetic benefits too. In the Ayurvedic texts, haritaki paste is recommended for the treatment of cracked heels, also known as 'padadari'. Therefore, a clinical study was undertaken to test this claim,

19

wherein 5 g of powdered fruit was mixed in 10 g of ghee and applied on the feet for four consecutive days. It was found that those treated with haritaki showed 'significant symptomatic relief in fissures of the heat, dryness and burning sensation'.

Another study conducted on 150 people found that haritaki consumed with honey during the spring season improved health and the overall quality of life. This is based on the Ayurvedic concept of ritu haritaki, wherein this herb is taken with various *anupanas*, or carriers, based on seasons. So, for spring, it should be taken with honey; during summer, with jaggery; in monsoon, with rock salt; during autumn, with sugar; in early winter, with ginger; and during late winter, with pippali (*Piper longum*, long pepper). In another trial, eighty-two people tried the combination of 3 g of its fruit with 1 g of rock salt taken with warm water early morning during the rainy season and found to be effective in reducing the severity of common cold, cough and fever. This is reflective of the fact that the fruit is considered to be a *rasayana*, meaning an anti-ager, which can be taken periodically to improve general health.

Application

The haritaki tree is considered to be the home of Hari, or Vishnu. Hara is also the name of Shiva, so it is considered to be incredibly sacred. The great news is that once established, this plant requires no special care, can survive in areas that are prone to drought and is also frost-resistant. There are various varieties of this plant, which can be grown all across India. Indeed, the nurseries of your area would have a haritaki that is suited to grow in your climatic conditions. In general, trees grown from seeds take longer to bear fruit as compared to those grown from cuttings, which bear fruit in five to six years.

Most Indians are familiar with this fruit, as we have been consuming it in triphala. But did you know that you can also consume haritaki churna on its own, especially if you're prone to constipation? You need to take half a teaspoon along with warm water every night. However, as with every nutraceutical, this too should not be consumed for more than three months. Haritaki is also wonderful as a pickle, which can be consumed all year with your meals to boost immunity and enhance digestion. In fact, just like we have been adding amla to our salads, why not add harad as well, though it does have a slightly bitter taste, so it makes sense to add it to brine or ferment it a little bit.

Haritaki Hair Paste

This recipe is from a small study based on a recipe from a traditional Ayurvedic book called *Chikitsa Manjari* by D. Sreeman Namboothiri. It is prescribed for a dry, itchy and flaky scalp.

Ingredients

30 g haritaki powder
30 ml buttermilk

Method

Mix both ingredients and apply to the scalp for seven consecutive days to improve scalp health. Wash off with plain water and do not use hair oil during this time.

SANDALWOOD, AGARWOOD AND HALMADDI

The trio of sandalwood, agarwood and halmaddi—the woods of worship—have been used across cultures for centuries. The earliest mention of plant aromatics such as these woods and resins in India was in the Rig Veda and the Atharva Veda. While it is common knowledge that sandalwood holds an exalted position in Indian homes and temples, not many are aware of other woods such as halmaddi and agarwood (oudh), which are equally revered for their psycho-spiritual benefits. You may not be aware of halmaddi by its name even though you are familiar with its 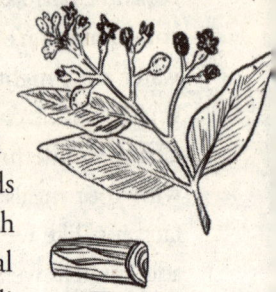 sweet, wet fragrance that wafts through the temples of south India. It's a resin from the Ailanthus triphysa (also Ailanthus malabarica) tree, which is also known as the Malabar tree of heaven, and is used to make matchsticks, as it burns very well.

This fragrant resin was commonly used in Nag Champa incense along with frangipani. Contemporary Nag Champa incense, however, does not contain this resin any more due to the incessant use and destruction of this tree, which led to the ban of leasing halmaddi trees in the 1990s. Decades later, in 2011, when more than 50,000 trees were leased out by the Mangalore Forest Division, there were reports of clear violation of rules which saw even young trees being incised to extract the resin. This unabated usage of fragrant woods, especially sandalwood and halmaddi, has made them almost endangered.

Oudh, of course, has worldwide recognition because of its use as a fragrance. But did you know that it is known as the 'Wood of Gods' and is revered in Hinduism, Christianity, Islam and Buddhism? Agarwood has been mentioned as a fragrant product in Sanskrit texts way back in 1400 BCE. In 65 BCE, Pedanius Dioscorides, the Greek physician, botanist and pharmacologist, described its application in medicine and the earliest recorded plantation of agarwood by humans goes back to 300 CE in China. Like sandalwood, oudh too remains fragrant over a very long period of time as long as it is handled properly—exposure to sunlight and heat can vitiate its fragrance, which is why it is valued as a commodity. There is, in fact, evidence of agarwood trade between Southeast Asia and China, Japan, the Middle East and India.

In Sanskrit, agarwood is known as aloes, agaru or aguru, which means non-floating wood. In China, it is known as chen xiang, the sinking incense, as it is derived from a wood that sinks underwater. The Hindi word 'agarbatti' for incense stick is derived from the word 'aguru'. This wood was synonymous with wealth and status. In fact, both oudh and sandalwood also find mention in the epic Mahabharata, especially describing the amphitheatre outside King Drupada's capital which was 'enclosed on all sides with high walls and a moat, scented with black aloes and sprinkled all over with water mixed with sandal paste and decorated with garlands of flowers'. The use of fragrance is a huge part of Buddhist traditions. Agarwood was one of the ritual deposits found within the cavity of the

486 CE bronze sculpture of Buddha Maitreya. Additionally, it is widely known that Prophet Mohammed preferred the scent of oudh over all other fragrances.

As for sandalwood, we know that it is one of the oldest fragrances in the world, with the earliest mentions going back to 200 BCE in the *Milinda Panha* and 100 BCE in *Patanjali Mahabhashya*. It is believed that Lakshmi, the goddess of wealth and abundance, lives in the sandalwood tree, which is why it is also known as Srigandha, Sri being another name for Lakshmi. It is also believed that Goddess Parvati created her son Ganesha, the god of new beginnings, with the paste of sandalwood and turmeric. This wood has spiritual significance in other cultures as well. For instance, it is used in the sacred fires by Buddhists and Zoroastrians, as it is believed that this soothes the troubles of humanity. Even the Egyptians used it for medicinal purposes, embalming and ritualistic fires. Poet, artist and Nobel laureate Rabindranath Tagore said of the sandalwood tree: 'As if to prove that love would conquer hate, the sandalwood perfumes, the very axe that lays it low.'

The Science

Someone sent me a lavender body lotion the other day and as soon as I applied some of it on my hands, I immediately saw—in my mind's eye—my grandmother's face. The fragrance that I didn't consciously remember, but it brought back a memory with photographic precision. Nothing about this experience is unusual because it happens to all of us, but it was extraordinary indeed. Did you know that the phrase used to describe this type of experience is 'Proustian moment', based on Marcel Proust's famous line in his book *À La Recherche Du Temps Perdu*, in which he describes how a memory resurfaced in his mind on tasting tea-soaked madeleines.

Perhaps it's the proximity of our olfactory bulb to all the amygdala, hippocampus and other regions associated with fear, emotions and memory that makes smell such a potent governor of mood and memory. In fact, even taste is associated with our sense of smell. Without smell, there will be no taste. Perhaps the ancients knew this instinctually, which is why most of the sacred rituals were associated with sweet smells, which we now know affect us at both an environmental and cellular level. Take the case of sandalwood for instance. There was a small German study that found that the scent of sandalwood helps enhance wound healing. What's even more amazing is that it doesn't even have to be real sandalwood; synthetic sandalwood is equally effective.

The main therapeutic ingredient of sandalwood oil is α-Santalol (alpha-santalol), which has been found to 'remove negative programming from cells and increase oxygen around pituitary and pineal glands'. This is a good time to remind ourselves of the traditional practice of applying sandalwood tilak, bindi or *lepa* all over the forehead, as this application is believed to cool down the entire body. After all, the pineal and pituitary glands are located in the forehead. In fact, the absorption of sandalwood through the skin results in mental relaxation.

As for its skin benefits, in India, sandalwood paste has been used for centuries to calm and clear the skin. Studies have found that sandalwood oil helps protect the skin against oxidative stress caused by blue light and urban dust. Another study also found that 75 per cent of paediatric eczema/atopic dermatitis patients achieved a 50 per cent reduction in their Eczema Area and Severity Index (EASI) score with 'East Indian' sandalwood oil preparations. Indian sandalwood contains about 70–90 per cent α-Santalol and β-Santalol (Beta-Santalol) as compared to Australian sandalwood, which comprises 20–40 per cent of these active ingredients. Therefore, Indian sandalwood is far superior in terms of fragrance and therapeutic benefits. However, due to restrictive policies, it is unfortunate that Indian sandalwood is now an endangered species.

Halmaddi has a similar story, as it was named a protected species in the 1990s. The problem is the incessant harvesting of plant ingredients with zero foresight. The ancient Ayurvedic texts always spoke about the correct season, time and even *nakshatra*, i.e. the placement of the stars, to harvest or excavate natural ingredients. Today, this isn't so, as we destroy plants and natural resources with a singular focus: personal profit. This is why we are losing precious resources not just in India but around the world. While sandalwood is still popular and has a lot of studies supporting its benefits, one cannot say this is the case with halmaddi. In folk medicine, this has been used as an antidote to cobra bites, as well as to treat conditions such as asthma, typhoid and dysentery. As far as fumigation is concerned, its benefits have not been studied extensively although its extract has been found to have anti-bacterial effect and its bark contains chemical constituents, such as quassinoids and malanthin, which show promise as anti-amoebic, anti-malarial agents.

Of course, there is no dearth of research as far as agarwood is concerned since it is still a highly valued ingredient in both cosmetics and spirituality. It's interesting that this oudh essential has been found to have a hypnotic effect. In an animal study, its inhalation was found to shorten the time it took to go to sleep and prolonged the sleep cycle, as it induced a relaxed state of mind. The smoke of agarwood too has therapeutic benefits. In another animal study, it was found that the major component of high-quality (kynam) agarwood was chromone, which had sedative, anti-depressant benefits by increasing the levels of serotonin.

Interestingly, a healthy agarwood tree doesn't produce the fragrant resin. The formation of agarwood happens by what I call a 'trauma response' to injuries made by lightning, animal grazing, insect or mold attack. Because of these injuries, the internal part of the plant is exposed and it secretes this precious resin as a defence mechanism. This resin deposited around the wounds hardens around the tree over time and is used to make its signature aromatic oil. Unfortunately though, because of this response to stress, these trees have been manhandled by humans and is currently on the list of endangered species. This is why we need to treat all plants as sacred. Because when we do, we treat them with respect and reverence.

Application

All three plants are excellent for fumigation purposes or to utilize the essential oil for a sense of calm. I, however, am partial to the scent of halmaddi, with its sweet, damp fragrance that really lingers in the room long afterwards. Though it was commonly used in incense earlier, now there are very few places utilizing its fragrance. Still, there are a few brands that use halmaddi as part of its ingredients or simply use only this wood. You will have to look at the ingredients of an incense to verify its presence in the formulation.

Oudh chips are traditionally burnt in the same way as frankincense and myrrh; however, their use must be limited, as some studies have found that it may increase pollution and worsen asthma. Oudh is best used as an essential oil since its therapeutic effects can be enjoyed safely in the form of oil. Some believe that oudh oil works as an aphrodisiac, perhaps it's because of its association with luxury, however there is no scientific proof backing this claim.

Sandalwood can also be burnt as an essential oil and is an important component of a cooling Ayurvedic preparation called chandanadi, which is available as a tonic and hair oil, among other things. I do love the fragrance; however, I also like to use it as a face mask or lepa to be applied on the forehead for its cooling effect. Though there are various white sandalwood powders and sticks available in the market, it is difficult to find one that is authentic. The best way to find a good-quality white sandalwood powder is via the government-approved store in Mysore, where it is still better to buy a stick instead of the powder, which may or may not be adulterated.

While I was writing this book, I met a group of women in Chennai. Most of them had a sandalwood stick that had been passed down through generations, just like an heirloom. Whenever they wanted to use it as a mask or tika, they would freshly grind the stick and apply the paste.

How to Grind Sandalwood Paste

Ingredients

Sandalwood stick
Grinding stone
Water
An airtight jar

Method

- Choose a grinding stone that has a bit of texture to it. Pick one that's neither too rough nor too smooth. Keep it over a surface covered with fabric so that the stone doesn't move around while you rub the wood.
- Wet the surface of the stone with a bit of water. Don't make it too wet because you are looking for a slightly dense, not runny, paste.
- Then place the stick so that the entire length is in contact with the paste. Don't put the corner down but the flat surface so that the process is more stable and you get more paste.
- Keep adding ½ to 1 tsp of water and rub the stick till you get a paste.
- Transfer the paste to an airtight container and repeat the process.
- Repeat till you have the required quantity.
- Keep covered in the refrigerator for no more than a few days.

Sandalwood and Lodhra Face Mask

Ingredients

½ tsp sandalwood powder
½ tsp lodhra powder
A pinch of turmeric powder
Enough rosewater/milk/raw honey, all three to make a paste

Method

Mix all the ingredients together. Avoid milk if you have oily skin and honey if you have a heat rash. Apply the mixture and leave it on till it's semi dry. Then wash off, rubbing gently to exfoliate. Do not rub if you are on a skincare routine containing acids or retinol.

CANNABIS AND DHATURA

Although cannabis is classified as a narcotic today, it is known as 'joy-giver' and 'liberator' in the Vedas, composed almost 4000–5000 years ago. Another early mention of this plant was when it was listed as part of the Chinese emperor Shen Nung's pharmacopoeia. Emperor Nung, in fact, is considered to be the father of Chinese medicine. The common name for cannabis and hemp in China is 'Ma', which translated means numbness or anaesthesia. In India, we are aware that both cannabis and dhatura are considered to be the favourite plants of Shiva, the god of destruction, poison and medicine. The Ayurvedic name of cannabis is Vijaya, which literally means victory.

Cannabis has a long history of being used for 'peak experiences', which are defined by psychologist Abraham Maslow as spiritual experiences that feel 'unitive', 'transcendental' or 'psychedelic'. Though many herbs are used across the world, cannabis is the least potent, especially when compared to other entheogens, which are psychoactive substances, such as psilocybin or mescaline, that help us find the divine within. The Atharva Veda, in particular, mentions the usage of cannabis and the recital of magical hymns to control the elements of nature. This text hails *bhaang* as one of the five sacred plants and as a source of happiness, donator of joy and bringer of freedom. In Ayurveda, the cannabis plant has been highlighted for its *deepana* (digestive stimulant), *pachana* (digestive), *ruchya* (taste promoter), *madakari* (intoxicant), *vyavayi* (short acting), *grahi* (withholds secretions), *medhya* (memory booster) and *rasayana* (adaptogen) activities.

It is a well-known fact that sadhus utilize cannabis to achieve peak spiritual experiences. But did you know that even a sect of Sufis use hashish as a substance to heighten euphoria and deepen concentration. Cannabis became a part of Western medicine in the late 1890, when renowned British physicist John Russell Reynolds prescribed cannabis tincture to ease Queen Victoria's menstrual cramps. To create his tincture, he used cannabis from the same source so that he could standardize the recipe. This was because different varieties produce different effects, depending on the season and location of the plant. Toxicity can be unpredictable depending on the sensitivity of the patient to any of the various types of cannabis. After he secured it from a single source and created his tincture, it was administered with great care—just a few drops on a slice of bread or a piece of sugar—and the dosage would be increased slowly and precisely, if at all. He is known to have recommended the usage of cannabis indica in epilepsy, asthma, migraines and depression. He was quoted in *The Lancet* as saying, 'When pure and used carefully, (cannabis) is one of the most valuable medicines we possess.' In 1785, evolutionary biologist Jean-Baptiste Lamarck decided that the cannabis plant found in India was different enough—that it should have its own name, so he named it *Cannabis Indica L.*, which means cannabis from India. It is also known as Indian hemp.

In terms of medicine, dhatura holds an exalted position. However, be informed that though therapeutic, it must never be consumed as a hallucinogen or to self-medicate, as essentially all parts of this plant are poisonous. From poison comes most medicines; dhatura is no different. It has several uses in Ayurveda, homeopathy and modern medicine. In the Vamana Purana, there is a story of Samudra Manthan, churning of the ocean of milk, by gods and demons together to release the elixir of life. When the churning happened, the first thing to come out was the lethal Halahala poison, which was so strong that its noxious vapours killed both devas and asuras. To save the world, Lord Shiva swallowed this poison, which turned his neck blue, giving him the name Neelkantha, or the blue-throated one. The Halahala poison also gave birth to the dhatura plant, which grew out of Shiva's chest, making this poisonous weed especially close to his heart. Even today, on Shivaratri, the thornapple fruit of the plant is given as an offering to calm this ferocious god. Devotees believe that by offering dhatura flowers or fruit, they let go of toxic emotions, such as envy, anger, fear and cowardice.

The dhatura plant is also associated with dark mysticism, such as in the ancient tantric text, *Vajramahabhairava-Tantra*. In such ancient texts, several destructive spells are mentioned that make use of the dhatura wood and fruit, whether to separate a couple, to drive someone insane, to turn wealth into poverty or for instant death. The earliest mentions of this plant were in the *Arthashastra* and *Kama Sutra*. In *Arthashastra*, it is mentioned in section duties of the superintendent of liquor, listed as one of the several plants that give liquor a heady taste. Dhatura has another fierce association, as it is also the headdress of Nataraj, Shiva's avatar who performs the Tandava Natyam, or the dance of destruction.

Even in the tribes of North and South America, the dhatura plant was taken for purposes of divination, communication with spirits of the dead or contact with supernatural guardians. There are several indigenous myths which speak of the usage of dhatura as a stabilizing factor. In some tribes, it was given to men to make them more masculine and to women so that they become more courageous. One myth being that if a woman consumed dhatura, she would not be attacked by a bear while foraging. Rattlesnake and grizzly bear were believed to be vicious because they stay away from the dhatura plant, which has a stablilizing effect. In the Chumash tribe, which belonged to an area we now know as California, the one who went to collect this plant purified himself by abstaining from alcohol, meat and grease for a few days. When he approached the plant, he prayed first to the dhatura spirit and respectfully sought permission before gently unearthing a root of the plant and then covering up the hole. But this was also the time when animals and plants were considered to be as important as people—they were precious entities that were nothing less than sacred.

The Science

The cannabis plant has been popular for thousands of years, but its popularity fluctuates with legal policies. Today, it is considered to be the panacea of health. But in India, the flowers (gaanja) and resin of the flower (charas) are classified as a narcotic since the government passed the Narcotic Drugs and Psychotropic Substances (NDPS) Act, 1985, banning the cultivation, production and consumption of cannabis. This was because it was regulated and prohibited in the US and Europe, and we passed this after signing the UN's Single Convention on Narcotic Drugs. However, the other parts of the plant, namely, the leaves (bhaang), the seeds and the fibre are outside the purview of the NDPS Act. Therefore, while holding just a small amount of gaanja or charas can get you arrested, bhaang, an edible preparation used in drinks and sweets, is legal.

The irony is that as this weed was razed from our roadsides where it grew wild, the West legalized it and now cultivate and consume it, giving rise to a billion-dollar industry where India, the land of hemp, barely has any stake.

But there is one important yet ignored benefit of hemp cultivation, which is its effect on the soil. It is known that soil all over the world is now contaminated with heavy metals, pesticides, industrial waste, sewage, etc. Metals and other contaminants don't degrade but alter from one state to another. Phytoremediation can be enhanced with the use of industrial hemp (cannabis sativa), as the plant has the ability to extract metals and other contaminants from the soil with its deep, wide spread of roots. We know this process is successful because it was employed to remove contaminants from agricultural land around Chernobyl, Ukraine, after the nuclear disaster of 1986. In 2008, at a farming region in Italy that was contaminated by a steel plant, hemp was cultivated to leach pollutants, particularly dioxin.

Since these toxins accumulate in its stalks and leaves, they're not consumed as food or mixed into cosmetics. Instead, they are used for building material such as paper, cloth and even as biofuel. What's more is that hemp is a very fast-growing plant. Today, reforestation is one of the best strategies to reduce atmospheric carbon, therefore its cultivation is even more important. Climate scientists propagate the cultivation of fast-growing, short-rotation forestation for carbon reduction and as a source of biomass fuel. Additionally, it's also an excellent cash crop not only because it can grow quickly but also because every part of a hemp plant can be utilized to make oil, milk, cloth, paper, cosmetics, food and fuel.

Hemp and cannabis look similar since they belong to the same species, but they are a little different because cannabis contains more than .03–1 per cent tetrahydrocannabinol (THC). Therefore, cannabis or marijuana is responsible for the more narcotic and/or medical preparations. However, the most powerful medicines are made from narcotics, for instance opioids from opium. Cannabis is no different. Today, it's being researched for its therapeutic role in the management of sleep, pain, nausea and epilepsy. The data still doesn't show significant results, even though there is empirical evidence surrounding these potential benefits. This is not to say that Cannabidiol (CBD) and THC don't have a place in the future of medicine, but more research is required to understand its precise benefits. But what we do know is that the long-term use of marijuana impairs cognitive function, therefore as a substance it must be controlled. However, to abolish its presence from its natural habitat is like throwing the baby out with the bathwater.

Dhatura too is banned in India and for good reason, except for use in Ayurvedic medicine. Every part of this plant is poisonous, and ingestion—even in small quantities—can lead to convulsions, hallucinations, headache, coma in some cases and even death. But somehow, during Shivaratri, its presence is ubiquitous outside temples, as it is considered a favourite of Shiva. Be careful not to plant it at home because of its high toxicity. Instead, look for Ayurvedic preparations and rituals that make this ingredient shine in its full glory.

In Ayurveda, dhatura-based preparations are prescribed especially for hair. In a short-term study done on twenty-five people, it was found that the application of dhatura patra swarasa lepa, which is a concoction prepared from the juice of its leaves, all over the scalp for thirty days showed significant improvement in alopecia areata patients. There was relief in all parameters: 75 per cent reduction in hair fall, over 88 per cent reduction in dandruff and 80 per cent less itching, with over 60–90 per cent improvement in terms of reduction of dryness, foul smell and burning sensation. Although a small study, it shows that dhatura holds promise as an ingredient/component in hair products.

Just like hemp, dhatura too can be used in bioremediation, a process whereby hyper accumulator plants, which have the ability to absorb contaminants, are used to clean the environment. In one study, dhatura was used to remove TNT (part of explosives) from the soil by root uptake and also enrich the soil with microbial activity. When used in soils with levels up to 1000 PPM (parts per million), the plants still grew well with moderate levels of stress at high levels of contamination. The result was that 'TNT levels in the soil reduced to less than 10% in two weeks', making this a great option to clean the land around military bases and war zones. In another experiment, the stems and leaves of wild dhatura plants around the contaminated industrial area of Bhopal were collected to test levels of heavy metals. The tests showed that the plants had high levels of heavy metals such as lead, nickel, cadmium and chromium, which reflects its potential as a phytoremediator.

Application

Both these plants lie in the dark or grey area as far as usage is concerned. They are easy to grow and while cannabis is not poisonous, it is a prohibited resource. Dhatura, on the other hand, can easily be misused. Therefore, its cultivation must be done carefully. Nevertheless, the environmental benefits of both these plants hold a lot of promise, especially in our country, where large swathes of land are contaminated. These can be an inexpensive solution to improve soil quality. Hemp has a deep root system, which also helps prevent soil erosion. Therefore, its cultivation along riverbanks and mountain slopes, where it grew naturally earlier, is imperative.

For personal use, there are many preparations of dhatura that you can try. As dhatura's potential in haircare is well documented in Ayurveda, one can try the traditional hair oil called dhurdhurapatradi, made out of this poisonous herb. This Ayurvedic tailam, which is a concoction of various herbs cooked in a base oil, is specifically targeted for dandruff and seborrheic dermatitis. As for cannabis, it is legal now to take it for medical conditions such as pain relief, anxiety and sleeplessness. One of the side effects of long-term marijuana use is paranoia; however, when taken as CBD with negligible amounts of THC, it doesn't lead to this. When you're choosing a variety of CBD oil, take care to choose one that is sourced from good-quality organic soil. As you now know, hemp or cannabis tends to absorb metals and other contaminants from the soil, therefore the source of CBD is immensely crucial.

Second, while choosing CBD, look for a full-spectrum oil, which has the full range of cannabinoids and terpenes that give the plant its healing powers. As compared to CBD isolate, which contains no other CBD compounds, broad spectrum has a wider range of benefits. Broad-spectrum CBD products are excellent for mental well-being and full-spectrum THC products are great for pain management. Still, if you're a beginner, it may be preferable to go with a pure CBD oil to test the waters and then choose a broad-spectrum organic CBD oil. Follow the dosage carefully: not a drop more than prescribed by the doctor.

Some people like to take CBD oil sublingually, which is to administer it under the tongue. This method shows the quickest results, but the effect doesn't last as long. However, more CBD is absorbed with this method. To do: take the prescribed amount and hold it under your tongue for 30 seconds and then swallow it. Do not eat or drink anything for about 30 minutes before and after taking CBD. The other way is to take CBD with a healthy fat, such as milk or ghee, to improve its absorption.

Ultimately though, with great power comes great responsibility. In the case of powerful plants such as cannabis and dhatura, this holds especially true. How can we utilize the power of these plants without falling into an addictive cycle? The key is restriction and control but not eliminating these valuable, indigenous species entirely, as it would be remiss not to use them for their environmental and medical benefits.

Bhaang Ki Chutney

Ingredients

90 g bhaang (hemp seeds)
5–6 cloves of fresh garlic
2–3 green chillies
Fresh coriander or a handful of coriander seeds
A handful of fresh mint leaves
Juice of one medium-sized lemon
Water as required
Salt to taste

Note: Besides the above-mentioned ingredients, some people also add other ingredients, such as roasted tomatoes, dry red chillies, fresh onion and cumin seeds, to adjust the taste and consistency according to their preference and palate.

Method

- Heat a pan. Dry roast the hemp seeds and keep aside.
- On a *sil batta* (*batan* and *una*, or grinding stone) make a paste out of hemp seeds, fresh garlic, green chilli, fresh coriander and mint.
- Transfer the paste from the sil batta to a bowl.
- Now squeeze the lemon juice and adjust the seasoning.
- Your bhaang ki chutney is ready and can be eaten with chapati, rice and fritters.

CINNAMON, CLOVES AND BAY LEAF

When it came to expeditions, nothing inspired sailors more than discovering the shortest route to find and harvest precious spices. The allure of cinnamon, cloves and bay leaf drove many explorers to the furthest corners of the earth, be it Christopher Columbus, who accidentally discovered America in the search of India, or Gonzalo Pizarro, who decimated jungles in Columbia, and tortured and killed indigenous people in the Amazon basin after he led a Quixotic search for the 'Land of Cinnamon'. It was only in 1498, when Vasco Da Gama made the momentous sea voyage to the Malabar coast that direct spice trade began between India and Europe. Before that, cinnamon was a part of fables, with traders creating tales of the mystical and ferocious Cinnamologus, Cinomolgus, or Cynnamolgus bird, which made its nest with cinnamon twigs. It was said that to forage the bark, this bird had to be given large pieces of meat, the weight of which broke the nest. Of course, this tale is false but was artfully crafted to horrify merchants and prevent them from seeking the direct source of this delicious spice.

So great was the allure of cinnamon that its origins were kept hidden. Some experts believed it came from Somalia, while others believe that it came from Egypt, when the truth was that this ancient spice mainly came from the island Sri Lanka, or erstwhile Ceylon. Since its origins were kept shrouded, the Romans failed to recognize cinnamon leaves when they came to India. Cinnamon holds biblical importance too, with this spice being a component of the anointing oil used by Moses. It was also used in Roman funerals, in the embalming of Egyptian mummies and even the Greeks used it in food and medicine.

Cloves too have a rich history of mysticism and folklore. During Navratri, the festival celebrating the nine forms of Goddess Durga, cloves are given as an offering to the goddess to ward off evil eye and to invite success and joy. They are also seen as a token of protection. During Christmas, oranges are often studded with cloves and hung with a ribbon as a symbol of good luck. The earliest mention of clove is from ancient India, where it was known as devakusuma, meaning the divine flower. It was also essential for visitors in the 200 BCE Han Dynasty to keep cloves in their mouth to freshen their breath before meeting the emperor. In Vastu Shastra, cloves are usually burnt with camphor to purify the air of the house.

In a similar vein, bay leaf too is considered to have protective qualities and to improve psychic abilities. It was used in the temple of Delphi, which was dedicated to the Greek god Apollo, where the bay tree is his emblem and sacred tree. According to local folklore, the oracle Pythia would chew bay leaf before uttering her prophecies. During those times, it was also believed that this tree offered protection from misfortunes and were therefore planted close to one's house. It was also believed that sleeping with bay leaves under the pillow increased artistic abilities, intelligence and psychic powers. Bay leaf is also used in Wiccan traditions to ward off negativity, to manifest desires and for protection.

What is it about these spices that gives rise to such folklore? Perhaps it's the pungent smell and flavour due to their potent phytochemical profile, which make them precious in culinary, medical and ritualistic practices.

The Science

The strong flavour of spices, or herbs for that matter, is very telling of their therapeutic properties. The stronger the flavour, the more complex is its antioxidant and phytonutrient profile. In fact, clove extracts were found to have the highest antioxidant activity. Additionally, cinnamon and clove were found to be among the spices with the highest phenolic content. But just because they have a high antioxidant profile doesn't mean they should be overused. By making the flavours of these potent spices very strong, nature has ensured that we never overuse these natural healers.

Traditionally, in India, we use spices in our foods giving us a balanced profile of nutrients. Still, many Indians suffer from poor health despite our diverse menus. This is because of a few reasons: one is because of a change in our diet, where we eat more refined foods and trans fats than ever before, secondly because of soil contamination, thirdly because of the overuse of spices. Of course, the number one reason for using these ingredients is to add flavour to our food. However, the secondary function of spices is to work as preservatives. To extract the flavour, we temper them in hot oil or ghee. Alternately, we roast them and then use them in curries. In both these techniques, the spices are allowed to 'bloom' and release their flavours.

Lately though, spices have taken centre stage as nutraceuticals, given the rise of lifestyle-related diseases and new information regarding the antioxidant profile of our potent masalas. But for every nutraceutical, the right source is incredibly important. For therapeutic purposes, the Ceylon cinnamon is preferred, as it contains low to negligible amounts of coumarin, a phenolic substance that is part of cinnamon. Coumarin has been connected to liver damage and is also recognized as a carcinogen. In terms of appearance, the Ceylon cinnamon is soft, lighter in colour and has several layers, whereas the regular cinnamon is hard, dark and rolled into a single layer.

The therapeutic benefits of Ceylon cinnamon have been well studied, especially in the case of diabetes and neurological diseases. For instance, half a teaspoon of it can help reduce blood glucose levels in type-two diabetes. It also helps by imitating insulin, thereby helping metabolize sugar in the bloodstream. It also helps reduce triglycerides and LDL, also known as bad cholesterol, along with cholesterol in general. Additionally, it has anti-blood clot properties as well. Ceylon cinnamon bark has also been found to be effective against the progress of Alzheimer's disease. It also showed promise in Parkinson's disease in an animal study, where it helped reverse biochemical and anatomical changes.

While both clove and cinnamon are great ingredients to enhance oral health, it has been found that cinnamon oil is more effective in eliminating bacteria and shows some potential in controlling oral candida. It is the time-tested method for dental health, having been used to check tooth decay in China since the third century BCE. Therefore, a combination of both is best. Clove has been a part of folk recipes for centuries around the world. Fried cloves mixed with honey is given to control vomiting, while chewing a clove with a few grains of salt helps soothe throat irritation.

Interestingly, clove oil has been used as a preservative in freshly cut vegetables, such as lettuce. It was found that when diluted clove oil was sprayed on the leaves, it helped control browning of leaves, reduced bacteria and improved the overall quality of the produce. Clove oil can also be used as a preservative in leafy green vegetables and can be applied as a preservative pre- or post-harvest. This is because eugenol, its active agent, is found to inhibit a variety of food-related bacteria and fungi. It also works well as an insecticide, which is why many families in India use whole cloves, along with neem leaves, as natural insect repellents when they store clothes.

For everyday use, clove is a miracle spice and for a reason. It has been found that just a drop of clove oil is 400 times more powerful as an antioxidant than blueberries. It has been found that eating just one or two cloves per day leads to improvements in blood sugar, insulin, cholesterol and triglycerides. But even though it has myriad benefits, it should not be consumed mindlessly. In Ayurveda, clove is considered to be heating in nature, therefore it is not advisable to consume it in summer or for people who are high *pitta*, meaning prone to acidity, rosacea, etc.

All spices seem to have a stabilizing effect on blood sugar and cholesterol. Bay leaf is no different. There are no major studies done on bay leaf and its effect on humans. It has been found that how we use bay leaf significantly alters its benefits. When bay leaves are infused in tea, there were no remarkable changes, but increasing the dosage is key. About 1–3 g a day of powdered leaves for 30 days can lead to a notable decrease in fasting glucose and triglycerides. But when the doses were increased to 10 g (administered in cookies), there was a significant decrease in the same parameters. Of course, eating high quantities of spices is definitely not advisable. With their potent, antioxidant-rich oils, it is better to consume them in small amounts during the right season.

Application

Spices aren't just used to add flavour to our food, they also purify and energize the house. Bay leaf especially has ritualistic significance and is known to be popular in Wiccan and pagan rituals. Of course, the energy of an atmosphere cannot be measured in concrete terms, so there is no conclusive data on its use in folk and religious customs. But an animal study did find that bay incense may improve memory formation and did effectively diminish a certain type of cognitive deficit. This proves that there may be some benefits behind these rituals.

Of course, the high antioxidant value of these spices means that they are prized in the beauty and wellness industry. They are often used in fragrances to bring warmth and complexity, mixed into tisanes for their healing powers, and utilized in cosmetics for their anti-fungal and antibacterial effects. Cinnamon-infused gel, for example, helps reduce inflammation, redness, plus the number and size of eruptions in mild to moderate acne. Clove oil too helps diminish bacteria that cause acne, while bay has been traditionally used in hair tonics. Still, if one has to experiment with these potent spices, they must be used as part of cosmetics than

DIY masks and oil, which could, if the percentage is wrong, end up burning your skin.

Morning Cinnamon Infusion

Ingredients

A stick of Ceylon cinnamon
Two mugs of water

Method

Boil and simmer two mugs of water with the Ceylon cinnamon stick till the water evaporates and reduces to one mug. Drink this water before breakfast to reduce inflammation and to get an antioxidant boost.

Abundance Ritual with Cloves

This ritual should be performed on a new moon day or in a waxing moon phase to create the energies of growth and beginnings.

Ingredients

Bay leaves (symbolic of success and wealth)
Cloves (known for attracting prosperity and protection)
A fire-safe bowl or cauldron
Matches or a lighter

Preparation

Set Your Space: Choose a quiet time, when you will not be disturbed. Clean the area where you will perform the ritual, physically and energetically, to welcome new energies.

Intent Setting: Take a moment to clearly define your intentions for this ritual. What type of abundance are you seeking? Is it financial abundance, good health, love or a combination of all? Write your specific intention on a bay leaf using a marker if you wish to personalize your ritual further.

Method

- Assemble the Ingredients: Place a few bay leaves and a handful of cloves into your fire-safe bowl or cauldron.
- Lighting the Herbs: Carefully light the bay leaves and cloves, allowing them to catch fire. Once they start to burn, gently blow out any flames to let them smolder and release smoke.
- Chanting and Visualization: When the smoke starts spreading in the home, you may chant the given incantation to bring more energy and effectiveness in the ritual.

From deep down in earth and fire's might,
Summon my deepest wishes to light.

With clove and bay in smoke and blaze,
Call forth abundance in myriad ways.
Wealth and fortune, flow to me,
By my will, so shall it be.

- Smudge with Smoke: Gently spread the smoke around your body using your hand; start from your feet and move upwards to your head, visualizing the smoke clearing away all blockages to your flow of money and prosperity.

- Broaden the Ritual's Reach: Carry the bowl throughout your living and work areas, allowing the smoke to drift into every corner, closet and doorway. Let the smoke's presence infuse your entire space with the energy of abundance. Focus particularly on spaces where financial activities or business decisions take place.

- Conclude the Ritual: After covering all necessary areas with the smoke, return to where you started. Express your gratitude to the bay leaves and cloves for their support in this ritual. Let the herbs continue to smolder until they burn out naturally, or extinguish them safely.

- Dispose the Ashes: Once the ashes have cooled completely, bury them outside. This action represents planting seeds for future wealth. If you lack access to a garden, respectfully scatter the ashes in a natural environment.

SAFFRON AND CAMPHOR

The are many stories of how saffron found its way to Kashmir. One legend says that it was bought by the Persians in the fifth century BCE. Kashmiris claim that it was bought to India by two Sufi saints who gifted this golden spice to a village chieftain who helped them recover from illness. Even today, there is a shrine dedicated to these saints in Pampore. Yet another theory is that saffron was already in India, as it has been mentioned in old Kashmiri tantric texts. Centuries later, Chinese herbalist Wan Zhen wrote in the twelfth or thirteenth century, 'The habitat of saffron is in Kashmir, where people grow it principally to offer to the Buddha.' Indeed, at Shravanbela Gola, a town in Karnataka, even today the Bahubali statue is sprinkled ritualistically once every 12 years with pure Kashmiri saffron.

But no matter what its date of arrival in India is, the fact remains that it is one of the oldest spices known to man, as it was found inside a prehistoric cave in Iran and in 3000–5000-year-old fresco paintings in Santorini. Saffron finds mention in the Old Testament and the Tanakh, or Hebrew Bible, and in Persia, it was cultivated as far back as the tenth century BCE. Saffron wasn't just used as a dye and in medicine; it was also a symbol of wealth and luxury. It is believed that Cleopatra, the queen of the Ptolemaic Kingdom of Egypt, added a pinch of saffron to milk and used it to bathe before meeting a lover. The debauched Emperor Nero was welcomed with showers of saffron as he made his way into Rome. One of Alexander the Great's favourite cocktails was a mixture of wine and saffron, as he believed it would give him more power on the battlefield and in bed.

In a similar vein, camphor is steeped in history and ancient wisdom, but unlike saffron, which still holds its place as a rare and expensive spice, camphor has several synthetic knock-offs that made it a sooty polluting resin rather than an exotic luxury, which it was earlier. Nevertheless, its fragrance is still associated with divinity and purity, but there is no doubt that it needs to be revived in its purest form. In fact, many temples have dropped the usage of synthetic camphor because of its polluting effects and the harm it causes to one's health.

However, before the advent of commercialized camphor, the highly valued variety came from the Camphor tree (*Cinnamomum camphora*), or the evergreen karpura tree. So effective was its smell against microbes and pollutants that it was used as a fumigant during the Black Death as well as during outbreaks of smallpox and cholera. It was also considered valuable in perfumery and embalming. Because of its purity, in earlier times, camphor was edible and used in many culinary creations. According to *Vaidyak Shabda Sindhu*, an ancient book of dietetics and culinary art, camphor is called 'chandrabhasma', meaning moon powder. In ancient times, camphor was also one of the elements used to make paan. In the Tang Dynasty in China (approx. 600–900 CE), camphor was included in the recipe of the first sort of 'ice cream', which was made with fermented milk.

In India, camphor is closely related to the divine. In fact, Lord Venkateswara applied a dab of camphor (karpuram) on his chin to heal a wound after he was struck with a crowbar. It is a testament to the healing and cooling powers of real camphor. Of course, for Indians, its menthol-like fragrance is quite familiar. It is found in temples, and we use it in diffusers, in havans and aartis during festivals. The Karpura Gauram Karunaavataram mantra clearly reflects its exalted place in worship. When translated, it means: One who is pure white like camphor, who is an incarnation of compassion, who is the essence of worldly existence, whose garland is the king of serpents, always dwelling inside the lotus of the heart. I bow to Shiva and Shakti together.

The Science

Saffron is indeed very precious since only the stamen of the saffron flower is used to make this decadent condiment. About 150 flowers are required to make 1 gram of this dried spice, which is why it is justifiably one of the most expensive ingredients. As an ingredient, it benefits us from the inside out: as a medicine, beautifier and flavouring agent. The bioactive compounds in it are safranal, crocin and picrocrocin. It has an antidepressant effect, and according to studies, it was found to be more effective than a placebo and equivalent to doses of imipramine and fluoxetine. It has also been found to prevent memory impairment caused due to chronic stress. It works by modulating the levels of certain chemicals in the brain, most notably serotonin. More sound data is required to prove its benefit as an antidepressant, but there is no doubt that it can be tried as an adjunct therapy to support other medicines.

The other benefit of saffron has been demonstrated in cases of glaucoma, where it was found that consuming saffron extract led to a reduction in eye pressure. Additionally, this spice was also studied for age-related macular degeneration, where it was found that consuming saffron for three months helped improve retinal function and after six months, it helped reduce macular thickness. Therefore, it may be considered as a supplement for those with eye problems.

Additionally, the application of saffron extracts has benefits for the skin too, as it has been found to inhibit tyrosinase, which may increase pigmentation, and helps synthesize collagen and hyaluronic acid. Of course, there are also studies to show it could possibly be an aphrodisiac for men as well as women, but these studies have mostly been inconclusive. Still, if you look at the mind-calming, pain-reducing, skin-brightening qualities of saffron, it could also be considered to be an aphrodisiac in an indirect sense.

Camphor used to also hold a similar position as saffron in earlier times, but these days, this ingredient is fraught with controversy, especially regarding toxicity when accidentally inhaled or consumed, especially by small children. One reason is contamination, second is incorrect usage and third is that most variants are made synthetically, which immediately cuts down its wellness potential. It has been found in animal studies that the natural form was non-toxic, whereas the synthetic form led to toxic effects and behavioural changes. Additionally, there's also the assumption that this is a

100 per cent safe substance, but it should not be within reach of animal companions and infants.

The truth is that camphor should be avoided by pregnant women and kept away from young children. Also, when using camphor for beautification and spiritual purposes, only the purest, most natural form should be utilized. Nevertheless, this ingredient is extensively used, whether it is in balms to clear a blocked nose, calm a headache or soothe irritations due to contact dermatitis. Camphor-based drugs have been developed for certain types of cancer and chronic inflammatory diseases. And of course, it is commonly used in both Ayurveda and unani medicine for its cooling, antiseptic and stimulating effects. Cineole, also known as eucalyptol, is one of its natural compounds. It is known to reduce inflammation, break up mucus and dilate the pathways in the lungs, which is why it was traditionally used to treat breathing disorders. Additionally, it has also been found that camphor could possibly decrease the production of nitric oxide. Since experiments have found nitric oxide to play a role in headache, an ingredient that inhibits its production can help control headaches.

Camphor is also known for its anti-microbial benefits, which is why it is possibly recommended for fumigation. The essential oil extracted from its leaves, flowers and twigs showed anti-fungal action against seven stains of fungus. Camphor has also shown fumigant toxicity against insects such as red ants, which makes it an excellent option to develop eco-friendly products to control pests.

Application

Both camphor and saffron are woven into the fabric of life in India. Saffron is diffused in our homes every day, burnt in temples, added to Ayurvedic oils, and even used to flavour sweets and paan. Because camphor has cooling effects on the skin, the easiest way to use it is to mix a small piece of edible camphor into a face mist or toner. Camphor cannot dissolve in water on its own, therefore it's essential to crush and then add it to the toner. You can also crush and mix it to a hair oil for its cooling and anti-microbial effect on the scalp.

The other way is to burn it using a diffuser. Just crush some camphor, add a few drops of water and burn it on an oil burner. The challenge, however, in using camphor is to learn to differentiate between natural and synthetic varieties. The best variety of camphor is Bhimseni, which is 100 per cent natural and edible. One way to know whether it's natural and pure is to immerse it in water: if it sinks completely, it is pure. Natural varieties also burn completely without leaving behind any residue except a gentle fragrance. The synthetic varieties will smell too strong, like a decongestant balm and be somewhat grey or brown in colour as compared to natural camphor, which is always white.

As for saffron, the one way to determine its purity is to observe how quickly it releases colour. Just add a pinch to cold water; if it colours the water quickly, the 'saffron' is artificially coloured. If it slowly releases a yellow/orange tinge, it is good quality. The threads of saffron are also trumpet-shaped, meaning wider on one side and then narrow on the other. When rubbed between your fingers, they should release a yellow tinge. Lastly, taste the saffron. It should be bitter in taste; if it is sweet, it's a sign of inferior quality.

Saffron Milk or Water

The therapeutic dosage of saffron is 30 mg, which amounts to 20–30 threads a day. However, traditional wisdom suggests 1–3 or 4–5 threads in winter, which is certainly better for long-term usage. Studies have found that saffron has a beneficial effect on the quality and duration of sleep because its compounds such as crocin and safranal induce hypnotic effects. In Ayurveda, the combination of saffron and milk is most effective because milk increases the bioavailability of this spice. Saffron yogurt has also been studied and it has been found that adding it to yoghurt increases its polyphenol content and antioxidant properties. Having said that, you can also take saffron with warm water or nut milk. For a bedtime drink, try this recipe.

Ingredients

100 ml warm milk (dairy or nut)
A pinch of nutmeg
2–3 stands of saffron
Rock candy (mishri) or honey to sweeten

Method

- Warm the milk but don't make it too hot.
- Add the saffron with nutmeg powder, which has been shown to aid sleep.
- Add raw honey for its warming effects in winter or rock candy, which is more cooling to sweeten during summer.
- You may skip the sugar entirely if you wish.

Saffron and Chironji Face Mask

Ingredients

1tbsp chironji (cuddapah almond) seeds
4–5 threads of saffron
A little bit of milk to soak the above

Method

Soak the ingredients overnight. Grind to a paste next morning (add more milk if necessary). Apply all over the face and neck. Rub off when semi-dry.

BRAHMI AND GOTU KOLA

There are so many herbs that are synonymous with each other in Ayurveda, but the most common ones are brahmi (*Bacopa monnieri*) and gotu kola (*Centella asiatica*), both of which are called brahmi. Of course, they are quite different from one another: bacopa grows in water and has small white flowers, whereas centella grows on soil and has circular leaves. Moreover, you'll find bacopa in a lot of hair oils, whereas centella is popular in skincare formulations, cica creams for instance.

What they have in common is an ability to cool the mind, which is why they are considered immensely sacred. Brahmi is named after Lord Brahma, the god of all creation and knowledge. Indeed, with its memory-boosting benefits, this certainly is an apt name for this miraculous herb, which was also supposedly used by Vedic scholars to memorize lengthy scriptures. Also known as 'the herb of grace', its powers are more enhanced when combined with other intellect-sharpening plants such as gotu kola, jyotishmati and/or shankhapushpi.

Gotu kola is known as mandukaparni, as the leaves resemble the feet of a frog, and also the Saraswati plant, named after the goddess of knowledge, who incidentally is the wife of Brahma. In TCM, it is known as the fountain of life. According to one legend, a certain Chinese herbalist lived for 200 years because he consumed this sacred herb. Today, gotu kola especially has seen a huge revival because of its calming effect on the skin, which makes it the main component of skin-soothing cica creams. Of course, it's the same cooling effect that calms the mind and reduces inflammation when consumed internally.

The Science

There is not enough conclusive evidence to show that brahmi on its own creates statistically significant changes in memory and cognition. However, there are small placebo-controlled studies on humans and several animal studies that reflect some benefit. Since it is recommended for memory, this herb has been tried on patients with Alzheimer's and other neurodegenerative disorders. But the most benefit it has shown on is healthy patients of all ages. In a study, sixty medical students were given 150–300 mg bacopa extract twice daily for a placebo for six weeks. In the dose of 300 mg twice a day, it showed significant changes in memory and cognition. The supplements also boosted the serum calcium levels in the brain, but within the range. Though calcium is popular for its strengthening effect on the bones, it also helps regulate several neural functions and memory.

In another study of seventy-six adults between the ages of 40 and 65, the results showed a significant effect of the herb on information retention. What's more is that during the follow-up tests, the rate of learning was not affected, which suggested that brahmi helps retain new information. Brahmi has sedative, nootropic (improving thinking, learning and memory) and adaptogenic (ability to handle stress) benefits

59

for the skin. A special extract of brahmi called CDRI-08 has been part of most of the trials. In one such trial for CDRI-08 and ADHD, it was found that the regular intake of this herb improves attention and cognition in adults.

Though gotu kola is an essential ingredient in skin-calming cica creams, it also has benefits for the mind. In animal studies, it showed potential in treating Alzheimer's. That the anti-inflammatory quality of gotu kola also helps calm the mind is no surprise. It has been found that this herb helps decrease TNF-alpha levels, which promotes inflammation. If you have high levels of TNF-alpha, it means that inflammation is going on longer than it's supposed to, for instance these levels are high in burn victims. Gotu kola helps decrease the levels in both mind and the skin to help lower inflammation.

Of course, the best way to consume nutraceuticals is by combining them. Bacopa and centella work beautifully together. But having said that, if you are on any anti-anxiety drugs or antidepressants, always consume these herbs after consulting your doctor. This is because they can have an adverse effect or reduce the efficacy of these medicines, as observed in some animal studies. Most of these herbs show promise in healthy adults and children. Anyone with a condition must stick to their protocol or consult a mental health professional.

Application

Whether as a tea, tonic, hair oil or in skincare, these herbs have shown many benefits. In India, brahmi is an essential component of hair oil. The Ayurvedic vaidyas were far ahead of the green beauty industry, understanding that the skin can absorb certain ingredients. This is why you will see all the herbs that are 'medhya', or brain boosting, are used in hair oils. For instance, bhringraj, jatamansi and brahmi, all are recommended for their calming, sedative properties and are an intrinsic part of Ayurvedic hair oil recipes. In fact, brahmi-infused medicated ghee or oil can also be used for nasya treatment, where you dip your little finger in the ghee and use it to coat the inside of your nostril.

Brahmi Amla Hair Oil

Ingredients

A handful of fresh brahmi leaves or a couple of tbsps of dried powder
½ cup of grated, fresh amla or 2 tbsp of dried powder
250 ml coconut oil
A handful of curry leaves
1 level tsp of fenugreek seeds
1 level tsp of camphor

Method

Heat up the oil but don't bring it to a boil. Then add all the ingredients, except camphor. Leave it to simmer for 5–10 minutes. Then leave the ingredient in the oil and cover till it cools down. Add the powdered camphor. Store in a glass bottle or jar. You may strain the oil, but I like to keep it with all the ingredients. If you want to enrich the oil further, cook it in an iron wok.

Brahmi and Gotu Kola Tea

Ingredients

1 tsp each brahmi and gotu kola powder
(If you're growing these herbs at home, then take about 1 tbsp each of the leaves.)
A pinch of mulethi to add a dash of natural sweetness

Method

Boil the ingredients together in 100 ml of water till it reduces a little bit. Strain and drink.

Brahmi Medicated Ghee

Ingredients

500 g ghee
½ cup of brahmi power or a cup of the paste of fresh leaves

Method

Heat the ghee and add the powder or paste. Let it simmer for half an hour. Transfer into a mason jar. Eating medicated ghee on an empty stomach is the best way to consume it. Wait till the ghee is digested, i.e. about an hour, before ingesting anything else. This recipe is perfect for summer because both brahmi and ghee are calming for the mind and body.

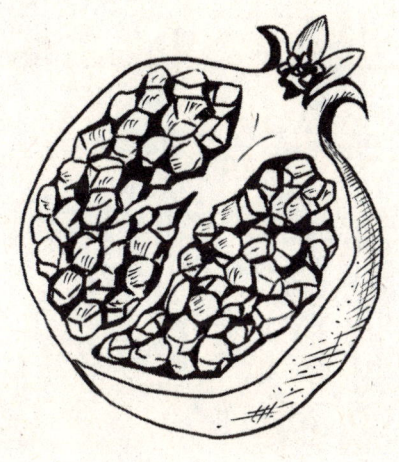

PART II

Surrender

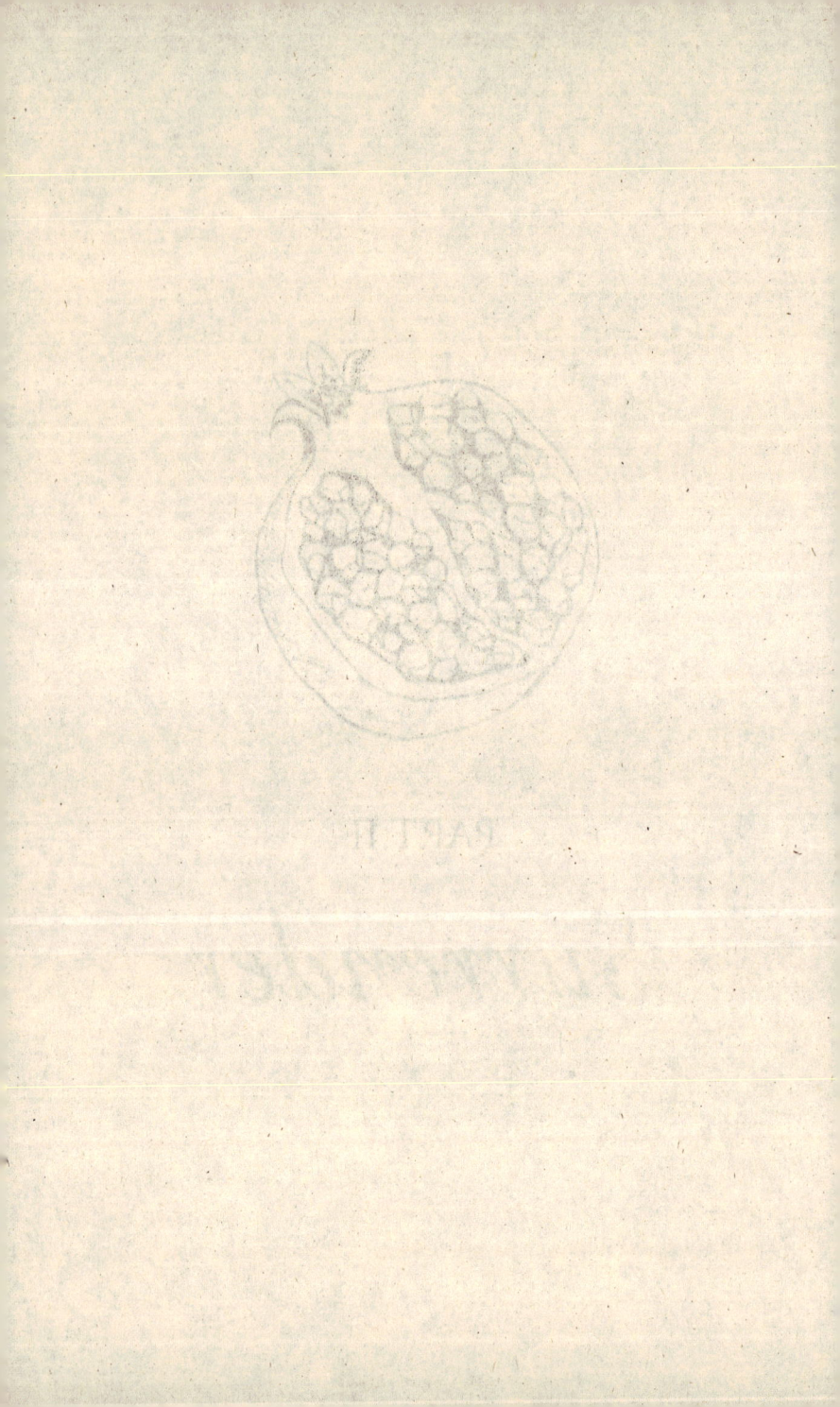

INTRODUCTION

To get close to the divine, one must surrender all forms of control and embrace uncertainty. As difficult as that may sound, it is important to remember that the most rewarding experiences in life are the ones we don't expect. Today, we know that our life is a manifestation of our inner desires. While on the one hand, it makes us feel powerful and in control over our destiny, on the other hand, we waste too much energy in trying to manifest a particular outcome. There are several problems with this. First, most of us don't know what we want, second and even more dangerous is knowing what we want, because what we want may not be good for us. Therefore, instead of wasting time and energy trying to manifest the future, it is best to surrender to the present and let life unfold naturally, slowly revealing delightful surprises and agonies like jewels lighting up the journey of life.

The concept of prasad—an offering of food, water or flowers to a deity—is a surrender of one's own ego before the divine. Every deity is said to have a favourite flower or fruit, which reflects their own inherent qualities; for instance, red flowers to the goddess that signify the bloom of womanhood. But look a bit deeper into these holy offerings and you'll find that these fruit and flowers are a gift for humanity itself. With properties that help calm the mind, fortify the body, detoxify and nourish, these sacred plants range from the garden variety to rare and exotic, but that doesn't make one superior over another. Additionally, just because a certain plant is considered sacred doesn't make it more special because all types of vegetation is a creation of the universe and each has a symbiotic relationship not only with each other but also with every insect, animal and human.

Part II outlines aromatic plants, fragrant flowers and ripe fruits that have benefits rooted in science. Whether it's making a paan and offering it as *dakshina* (donation), sacred berry trees that line places of worship, celestial flowers that are a favourite of gods and goddesses, and grains that are offered to the divine, these ingredients were special in the past and hold this place of significance even today. Each chapter contains recipes and rituals that will help you utilize these plants in your culinary, beauty and spiritual routines, reviving ancient traditions and rooting these ingredients to contemporary living.

As seekers continue forward on the spiritual journey, it is important to realize that to grow, surrender is essential. So give up expectations, the need for control and being invested in the outcome, as that is the ultimate act of faith. Release the show of strength and hyper independence and ask for help. There is something very beautiful about surrender because it has the potential to bestow us with so much peace. We spend too much energy in trying to control people and situations that in today's world, where we live continuously in fight or flight mode, to let go is the greatest act of defiance.

PAAN AND MISWAK

The betel leaf, or paan, is also called the 'green gold' of India because of its high economic value. It is a perennial, evergreen cash crop. It is a part of every Indian wedding, puja and festival, and it has been used and relished by us for thousands of years. In Hindu mythology, it is believed that Arjun, the warrior king, stole the paan vine from heaven and planted it on earth. Through time, it has consistently maintained its popularity as a mainstay in culinary and cultural experiences. It is mentioned in texts as old as the Vedas, as well as in Ayurvedic texts and Jataka Tales. It also finds mention in Mughal history and historical records of the British.

Of course, paan as an offering is a symbol of luxury, love and honour. It is mentioned in the *Kama Sutra* as an aphrodisiac, and as a part of the *solah-sringar*, which is the sixteen-step beautification process, the passing of paan between lovers is a transition to sex life. The sweet, fragrant quid of the betel leaf with rose jam, areca nut and slaked lime was used to refresh the breath and taken from one mouth and placed into another. According to Acharya Vagbhata, the ancient vaidya, paan should be taken in the morning, after a bath and after a meal. There was also a paan 'hierarchy' suggested by him. In ancient times, during ceremonies, the king received thirty-two leaves, the zonal officer twenty-four and a son-in-law eighteen leaves. Paan held an exalted position in Indian customs, as it was believed to improve the quality of voice, enhance digestion and sweeten the breath.

During the Mughal period, the betel leaf and nut became an important part of festivities and customs. So immense was its popularity among the *zenana* (the part of the house in which the women and girls of a family are secluded) that Princess Jahanara Begum was given the revenue of Surat by Shah Jahan to continue with her paan-related expenses. Historians have written that paan was as popular in India as coffee was in Turkey. Poet, musician and scholar Amir Khusro, who was also known as the father of Urdu literature, has called it 'the finest fruit of Hindustan'.

As betel grew to be a sign of an elevated social status—that of kings, nobles and magnates—it became an important commodity. Because it became an integral part of the dakshina, or offering to priests, the paan quid and leaf were sanctified. It is believed that several gods such as Lakshmi and Shiva and Chandra (the moon) reside within the paan leaf. It is also believed that Yama, the god of death, resides in its stalk, which is why the stalk is always broken away and never eaten. Even today, paan is a part of festivals and ceremonies, especially weddings, where exchanging paan leaves is a symbol of honour and love.

Indeed, the chewing of these spicy leaves and other tree stalks has been a cornerstone of dental hygiene for centuries. Miswak is no different. Known as siwak and arak in Arabic and mastic in Latin, this tree holds an exalted position in Islam, where dental hygiene is considered to be a sign of faith. The usage of the miswak stick to clean the teeth is a sunnah—practice of the Prophet himself—and therefore considered sacred. The Prophet is believed to have said in one of the hadiths, or prophetic traditions, that 'siwak purifies the mouth and pleases Allah'. In fact, offering namaz after using miswak is considered to be seven times more effective than performing without.

Traditionally, it is recommended that a miswak stick shouldn't be thicker than a finger. It should be made from bitter wood, for instance that of the peelu tree or miswak tree. The bristles should be soft since hard bristles are believed to cause a gap between the teeth. Ideally, the stick should be fresh, however an old stick can be refreshed by soaking it in plain water or rosewater for about 15 minutes. Cut the bristles of the stick daily. Miswak has also been mentioned in classical Arab poetry where it's symbolic of white teeth and a fragrant mouth. Abu Bakr Al-Razi, who is considered to be one of the greatest figures in the history of traditional Islamic medicine, said that this humble stick is good to freshen the breath, polish teeth, remove plaque and strengthen gums.

The Science

In recent times, the consumption of the traditional paan has been demonized and with good reason. Additions such as tobacco, slaked lime and catechu nut have been proven to be carcinogenic. However, betel leaf in itself contains cancer-protective properties. The pungent flavour of this leaf is indicative of the presence of potent polyphenols and it also contains vitamins such as beta carotene, Vitamin A, Vitamin C and Vitamin B. Among these bioactive components, hydroxychavicol, eugenol, chavibetol and chavicol show promise because of their chemotherapeutic or chemo-preventative benefits. Hydroxychavicol (HC), also known as 4-allylcatechol, is the major component and is shown to have anti-mutagenic properties. HC, in particular, has shown promise in inhibiting certain types of cancerous cells while leaving healthy cells unharmed.

Because of these powerful bioactive components and vitamin profile, the betel leaf also possesses anti-inflammatory, anti-fungal and germicidal properties. Because of this, it helps remove the foul smell of the mouth and helps improve digestion. Perhaps this is the reason why it has been used by Indonesian people for oral candidiasis. The chavicol present in the betel leaf is a potent antiseptic and chewing the betel leaves increases salivation in the mouth which, in turn, increases compounds and antibodies that help combat bacterial growth in the mouth. The leaf also contains a huge number of sterile molecules that are antibacterial in nature. Studies have shown that essential oil and extract from these leaves inhibit several fungal species, including candida albicans, and has also been found to control the growth of fungi that cause infections such as athlete's foot and ringworm infections. It works in synergy with other anti-fungal medicines and improves their effectiveness.

There are also reports that polyphenols in betel leaf extract are more than those in tea, which is why the betel leaf should also be looked at as a rich source of antioxidants. It also has anti-diabetic properties, which have been demonstrated in animal tests where blood glucose levels were significantly lowered with extracts of these leaves. It is unfortunate that these leaves have been demonized and are associated with poor oral health and bad habits. It is not wrong when this leaf is called the green gold of India because it contains fortunate benefits for long-term health. Eating a betel leaf but without slaked lime, areca nut or tobacco is indeed wonderful for health and is a ritual that is worth reviving in everyday life.

Application

The easiest way to incorporate this leaf in everyday life is to just include a betel and paan quid after a meal. However, this flavourful leaf can be added to desserts, salads and even smoothies. Use it to spice up your green juice or crush and stir it into a rose sherbet or thandai in summer.

The Healthy Paan

Ingredients

One betel leaf
½ tsp of fennel seeds
One clove
One cardamom
½ tsp of rose jam (gulkand, avoid if you have diabetes)
A couple of threads of saffron (optional)

Method

- Thoroughly wash the leaf. Wipe it clean and cut off the stem. Cut the leaves from the centre of the base, about an inch, so that you can fold it into a conical shape.
- Smear the leaf with gulkand. Over this sprinkle the fennel seeds, one cardamom and saffron.
- Then roll the paan into a conical shape and finally spear the paan together with the clove.
- Take your time to chew and enjoy the paan. Don't consume the paan quickly because the longer you chew it, the more the phenolic compounds get released and activated. So enjoy this as a ritual, not as a supplement that you have to gulp down quickly.

MANGO AND BANANA

When we think of sacred ingredients, we naturally assume them to be exotic and out of reach. But what is more sacred than everyday life and humble ingredients that nourish us from the inside out? Mango and banana are two ubiquitous trees that are utilized completely—whether it's the leaves, the fruits, the flowers or (in the case of mango) the wood. It's no surprise that these are a part of sacred rituals in India given their myriad uses. Mango of course is the king of fruits and is loved by everyone in India. Known as the fruit of the gods in the Vedas, mangoes were and still are symbolic of many things: devotion for the Buddhists, prosperity for the many kings who planted them along the pathways and also a symbol of love. Kama, the god of pleasure and love, has one arrow with a mango flower on it. The leaves are also associated with Lakshmi, the goddess of prosperity, and Saraswati, the goddess of knowledge. The evergreen tree is a symbol of eternal love and is therefore used in wedding ceremonies. The leaves are used to decorate entrances of homes as a form of a blessing, and along with the wood, they're also used in havans and pujas.

Of course, the taste of the mango fruit has held many powerful men in its sway. It is believed that the only thing Alexander the Great took back from the court of King Porus was a mango plant. Additionally, King Babur got so infatuated with mangoes that he decided to call India his home, just for the sake of this sweet fruit. Akbar is known to have planted about a lakh mango trees, called Lakh Bagh near Darbhanga, Bihar. The tree was popularized all over the world by famous travellers, such as the Persian poet Amir Khusro and Chinese traveller Hsuan-tsang, who waxed eloquent about this decadent fruit. The Buddhists were especially fond of mango, as they found it to be a ready fruit and associated it with Lord Buddha, who is said to have meditated under the shade of this magnificent tree.

The famous courtesan Amrapali, who was named after the mango tree, became associated with Buddha when she gave up her position as the royal courtesan to serve him. In fact, she also donated her mango orchards, Ambapali Vana, to Buddha, where he famously preached his Ambapalika Sutra. The mango tree is considered sacred because several sages, gods and goddesses are associated with it. The Ekambareswarar Temple (Ekambaranathar Temple) in Kanchipuram, Tamil Nadu, is where Parvati is said to have meditated under a mango tree. Miraculously, the 3500-year-old tree is still around. It is believed that if a person plants five mango trees, they will never go to hell.

Banana too is similarly revered and utilized thoroughly all over India. In fact, both the banana and mango tree are associated with fertility, perhaps because of being perennial. The banana plant isn't a tree but a large shrub. However, it is considered to be a tree because of its large size and is worshipped as one too. The entrance of a wedding pavilion is often festooned with two banana trees, as it is believed that these trees bring luck to the newlyweds. The tree is also considered to be Ganesha's wife as well as a symbol of Jupiter or Brihaspati and is therefore considered to be incredibly lucky when planted in one's home. Both bananas and mangoes are surrendered to the divine as offerings in everyday prayers. The fact that they're both commonly available and easy to grow makes them a worthy addition to any home and garden.

The Science

Things that are commonplace are sometimes ignored in terms of their nutritional value. Mango is known as the king of fruits, but it is assumed that this is because of its superior taste. The reality is that mango is also a panacea for health, as it contains a wide array of polyphenols and vitamins. For instance, it contains Vitamin C and beta carotene, which give it its yellow colour. Plus, it also has antioxidants such as quercetin, mangiferin, Gallic acid and coumarin. One mango, weighing about 210 g, gives 76.4 mg of Vitamin C, which is about 85 per cent of the required daily amount. It has been found that eating about 100 g of fresh mango daily increases the diversity of gut microbiome after four weeks, with the best results shown after twelve weeks. Eating this delicious fruit is associated with a higher intake of dietary fibre, magnesium, potassium, vitamins B_6, C and D, and choline, among other nutrients. Its pulp also contains pectin, which is an active component in apples and helps improve gut health and digestion. Additionally, it also contains amino acids, such as arginine, glycine, serine, leucine, isoleucine and alanine. Mango byproducts such as the seed and peel also have a considerable amount of fatty acid comparable with cocoa butter and must be looked at as serious contenders upcycled for use in cosmetics.

It's interesting that different varieties of mango have different levels of polyphenols and vitamins. The langara variety has the highest phenol content and antioxidant properties, whereas the ashwina variety had the highest amount of Vitamin C. The badami mangoes have the highest amount of citric acid concentration. Seventeen types of fatty acids have been identified with an increase in unsaturated fatty acids and Omega-3 and Omega-6 while ripening of Alphonso mangoes. Not to mention that this fruit is satiating for individuals with a sweet tooth, comparable to eating a dessert, which cannot be said for other fruits.

The other fruit that is extremely common is banana, which too is full of nutrients and excellent for the gut. In fact, the banana is another tree where every part can be utilized for something beneficial. The flower is eaten as a vegetable, the fruit is eaten as it is, the peel can be used in beauty recipes and hair masks, whereas the leaves are used as a platter to serve food. Banana has several bioactive compounds, flavonoids, phenolics, Vitamin E, ascorbic acid and enzymes. Raw bananas are rich in fibre and have high antibacterial activity. Bananas are a great source of carbohydrates, potassium, Vitamin B_6 and manganese. They also contain high levels of gut-friendly pectin. In fact, raw bananas are high in something called resistant starch, which works as a prebiotic, i.e., food for the microbiota in the gut. Banana peel is also rich in an amino acid known as tryptophan, which helps synthesize serotonin to elevate mood behaviour and cognition in the day and helps make melatonin, which helps us sleep better at night. In addition, banana pulp also contains serotonin, norepinephrine and dopamine, which gives us the feeling of well-being after we consume this humble fruit.

Application

The great news is that you don't need any special tips to make banana and mango a part of your everyday life. However, what is required is that we try to use as much of the fruit as possible. Overripe bananas are usually not consumed and are instead thrown away. Banana peels are always discarded as are mango peels and mango seeds. This creates the problem of pollution in the landfills, because they can emit greenhouse gases due to decomposition. Additionally, this wastage is also unfortunate because the peels and the seeds themselves are very rich in bioactive compounds. Of course, a lot of this must be controlled with robust industry practices, which prioritize upcycling of these ingredients. For instance, companies that make chutneys and jams out of mangoes can perhaps look at utilizing the seeds to create upcycled mango butter.

Bananas can be utilized in many ways. Unripe/raw bananas are being made into banana flour, overripe fruits are being used to make banana bread and the peel is used in tisane to help with sleep or even face and hair masks. DIY beauty recipes employ both overripe banana fruit and the peel, especially since the peels contain far more phenolic compounds and antioxidants compared to the fruit itself. Banana and mango peels can also be utilized to make a great organic fertilizer for plants, thus enriching the soil with potassium and other ingredients.

Banana and Honey Face Mask

Ingredients

Half overripe banana
1 tsp of raw honey

Method

With a fork mash the banana and honey together till it turns into a paste. Apply the paste to the face and neck. It might be a little messy, but the results will be worth it. Keep this on for 10 minutes to half an hour. Then clean the face/neck thoroughly with a damp washcloth or towel. This helps increase the hydration in the skin and heal its barrier.

Ripe Mango Curry

Ingredients

2 large or 4 small mangoes ripe, about 600 g before cutting

1 tsp salt

½ tsp turmeric

½ tsp red chilli, ground, or to taste

1 cup water, just enough to cover the mangoes in saucepan/pot

½ cup grated fresh coconut

½ tsp cumin seed

½ cup fresh plain yogurt

½ tsp mustard seed

8–10 fresh or dried curry leaves

2 whole dried red chilli

2 tbsp coconut oil

Method

- Dice the mangoes.
- Mix the mangoes, salt, turmeric and red chilli, in a 6" pot/saucepan. Bring it to a boil. Then lower the heat and cook for 15 minutes. Use a wooden spoon/spatula to mash the mango pieces as they cook.
- Grind the cumin and coconut in a mixie or grinder for about half a minute until well blended.

- Add the mixture to the mangoes and cook for another 2 minutes. Beat or whisk the yogurt until smooth. Add to mangoes and cook the curry for another 5 minutes on low heat. Do not bring to a boil.
- Heat oil in a wok or deep-frying pan on medium heat.
- Add mustard and curry leaves and stir. When the mustard starts to sizzle and pop, add whole dried red chillies and stir for about 2 minutes.
- Pour the tempered oil with the leaves and chillies (tarka) into your curry pot.
- Serve with hot rice.

Ela Ada (Rice flour dough stuffed with banana, coconut and jaggery)

Ingredients

1 cup rice flour
1½ cup water
½ cup fresh coconut, grated
1 steamed Kerala banana
¼ cup jaggery
1 tsp cardamom powder
2 tbsp ghee
5 banana leaf, pieces

Method

- Keep a pan on the gas stove with water and bring it to boil.
- Gradually add the rice powder to the water and mix using a wooden spatula/spoon. Once the mixture cools down, knead it with your hand to make a soft dough and then keep it aside.
- Combine the grated coconut, steamed banana, grated jaggery and cardamom powder with your hand.
- Take a piece of the banana leaf and place a lemon-sized dough in the centre of the leaf.
- Flatten the ela ada rice dough with wet fingers to get a evenly flattened dough. Fill the dough with 1 tsp of coconut jaggery mixture on one side of the flattened dough and fold from the other side and press lightly.
- Place the ela ada in a steamer/idli cooker and steam it for 10 minutes on high heat and then turn off the heat.
- Serve warm or at room temperature.

Banana Peel Tea

Ingredients

Leftover banana peels (preferably organic)

Method

You can make this tea in two ways. The first method would be to just save your banana peel of the day and at night slice it up and boil it in double the amount of water that you would drink. Strain and drink before bed.

The second method is to collect the peels over a week or a month and then freeze them so that they don't degenerate. Then you can dehydrate these peels in an oven till they're crispy. You can also sun dry them till they are completely dry and crisp. Then crush these peels and store them in an airtight jar. To make the tea, add 1 tsp of these dehydrated peels in a tea strainer in a cup. Then pour over boiling water, let it rest for a few minutes and then drink.

Aam Panna

Ingredients

1 kg raw mangoes
1 tbsp jeera
¼ tsp hing powder
A few sprigs of mint (dry or fresh)
Black salt as per taste
Khand (unrefined sugar) as per taste

Method

- Peel and boil the mangoes till they're soft and pulpy.
- Then remove the seeds and whizz in a blender with the water used for boiling. You may add more water if required, however it's better to make a more concentrated panna and then dilute while serving.
- Roast the jeera and hing and add to the pureed mango. Finish by adding mint, salt and sugar as per taste.

JUJUBE AND COCONUT

It's usually the humblest plants that are considered to be the most sacred. Jujube and coconut are no different. Jujube, or the humble Indian ber, is revered not only in Ayurveda but also in TCM. Interestingly, it holds an exalted place among Sikhs and their gurus preferred to plant it around gurudwaras. In fact, in Amritsar's Golden Temple, the Ber Baba Budha Sahib is an ancient jujube tree, considered to be more than 450 years old, named after Saint Baba Budha Ji. It is believed that praying to this tree and taking a dip in the waters of the Golden Temple can heal all ailments. This is just one among many historical trees that also include the Dukh Bhanjani Ber in Sri Harmandir Sahib and Lacchi Ber in its namesake gurudwara, where the fruits are the size of small cardamom pods. The Dukh

Bhanjani Beri tree also has folklore attached to it. As the story goes, the husband of Bibi Rajni, a woman who had great faith in the divine, was married off to a leper, who she took care of with great fortitude and love. As she carried him around all the holy spots in India, he was completely healed by taking a dip in a pond close to this tree.

Ber fruits are also offered to Lord Shiva, especially during Shivaratri. In fact, in the Panjvaktra Shiva Temple in the heart of Jammu, there is an ancient jujube tree under which Guru Nanak ji delivered a sermon and stayed for three days. Because of this, the tree is worshipped by devotees of Lord Shiva as a mark of respect for the saint who delivered his sermon in 1514. This ancient tree is also mentioned in mythological tales such as the Ramayana, where Shabari, an ascetic woman, tasted the ber fruits before offering them to Lord Rama. Indeed, this is just a testament to the ancient roots of this tree, which can be traced back to the Neolithic Age, almost 7000 years ago. The fruit is native to China but is now found in several other countries, as it has the ability to adapt to various soil types and temperatures. The fruit has been mentioned in the Chinese *Book of Songs,* which is more than 3000 years old. In fact, most varieties of jujube trees have mysticism associated with them. For instance, the Christ's thorn jujube (*Ziziphus spina-christi*), which grows in Africa, has been mentioned twice in the Quran. The traditional belief around this tree was that it was the host of certain saints and other spirits. Sitting under such a tree is considered to be lucky and the Prophet saw this tree in his visions of paradise. In Christianity, it is believed that this was the tree from which the crown was made for Jesus before his crucifixion. Indeed, such reverence across cultures just shows the value of this tree.

Another tree that is considered sacred is coconut, which grows along the tropics all over the world. In India, it is one of the trees that is called the kalpavriksha, which means the wish-fulfilling tree. The other kalpavriksha trees are parijat and banyan. The Malays call it 'pokok seribu guna', meaning the tree that provides all necessities. In the Philippines, it's called the 'tree of life' or the 'tree of heaven', whereas in Indonesia, it's known as the 'tree of abundance' because of its many uses. Interestingly, though most trees have been planted by people who take saplings or seeds from one part of the world to another, we have no role to play in the spread of the coconut tree. This is because coconuts can float over water for long periods and sprout when they reach the shore. In fact, there is a Tahitian folk song 'Niu-ola-hiki', which means 'O far-travelling coconut'.

There are many theories around the origin of the coconut tree. In Hindu mythology, this tree was formed when King Trishanku was thrown out of heaven by Indra. As the king was midair, Sage Vishwamitra held up the king with a pole, which turned into the trunk of the coconut tree; the head became the fruit and his crown became its fronds. In reality, archeological records reveal that the coconut tree has been around for 20 million years, predating our presence on earth. Old fossils found in New Zealand show that small plants like coconut grew there 15 million years ago. Fossils found in Kerala are even older, which is why perhaps there is folklore attached to this humble tree across all cultures in the tropics.

The tree is also supposed to be among the most useful trees in the world, which isn't a surprise, as it is used for its flesh, milk, oil and fibre. It is also used for a variety of purposes, from skincare and packaging to home décor, in the making of sporting equipment, agriculture, gardening and personal care. It's no wonder that the coconut is used in prayers and worship, given its significance in every aspect of our lives.

The Science

According to a classical book of TCM, the jujube was considered to be one of the five most nutritious fruits. It was also seen as medicinal, as it helped improve the quality of sleep, eliminate toxins and beautify skin, according to TCM. We now know that this humble berry contains seventeen minerals, including six macro elements and eleven trace elements, for instance vitamins A, B complex and C, along with calcium, magnesium and zinc. Additionally, these fruits contain at least a dozen major amino acids, whose presence varies depending on the variety of the fruit. In fact, one variety of this berry contains a whopping twenty-six free amino acids. Interestingly, micronutrients, particularly amino acids, are essential for sleep regulation, therefore it is not surprising that jujube is used in Chinese medicine for insomnia and has been used in China as a medicine to calm and soothe the nerves for about 1000 years. It's a commonly available, humble fruit, which holds immense potential to boost health and should be spoken about more, especially since it doesn't cost much.

The coconut is another humble local fruit that is a panacea for health. Especially in the last couple of years, coconut oil has seen a huge resurgence due to the popularity of the keto diet, which eliminates carbohydrates and sugars completely. Because of this, coconut oil, with 50 per cent medium chain fatty acids, can provide energy to a glucose-deprived brain. Additionally, this oil can help lower blood pressure and cholesterol and is seen as a potential Alzheimer's treatment as well. In my book *Glow* (Penguin Random House India, 2023), I have written that coconut oil and ghee are the only two fats that don't require bile from the liver to be digested and metabolized. Because of this, these fats are healthy for the liver and easy to digest. In *Glow*, I have also written that coconut water is very similar to the plasma we have in our bodies, which is why as soon as we drink coconut water, we instantly feel refreshed.

The coconut tree is also considered to be a type of kalpavriksha, which is supposed to be a wish-fulfilling tree. It is a fair description since it has numerous benefits. Coconut oil has antiviral and antibacterial properties because of the presence of lauric acid and coconut kernel is good for those with heart diseases and diabetes. The dietary fibre that is isolated from this kernel helps reduce cholesterol because of its hemicellulose component. Studies also show that tender and mature coconut water helps reduce the occurrence of lifestyle diseases. The flour, oil and milk made from this wonderful fruit possess antioxidant properties, while products made from its sugar are of low glycemic index. But that's not all. When the sap of this tree is fermented, it produces wine, vinegar and distilled spirits—this truly shows the utility of this common tree.

Application

Coconut and jujube are fairly easy to consume and are a part of everyday life. However, jujube has hardly reached the level of popularity as perhaps a blueberry. Therefore, efforts must be made to popularize this humble Asian berry at the same level as its Western counterpart since it holds immense potential for health and healing.

Soothing Coconut and Cucumber Face Mask

Ingredients

½ coconut (grated)
1 small cucumber (grated with peel and seed)

Method

Apply all over the face and neck and wash off after 20 minutes.

Avial

Ingredients

Cut vegetables evenly, 5-cm long and 1-cm wide.
4 drumsticks
50 g string beans
50 g elephant foot yam
50 g colocasia
2 unripe plantains
50 g cucumber
1½ tsp salt
2 tbsp curd (not too sour), whisked
1 stalk curry leaves
1½ tbsp coconut oil

Grind the following to a coarse paste:
1 medium-sized fresh coconut, grated
6 shallots, chopped
10 green chillies, chopped
1 stalk curry leaves
A pinch of cumin powder
½ tsp turmeric powder

Method

• Peel drumsticks, string and trim beans, and cut into
  5-cm-long pieces. Peel remaining vegetables and
  cut into 5-cm-long and 1-cm-wide strips.

- Place vegetables in a pan with salt and 1½ cup water and cook on high heat for 20 minutes till tender.
- Stir in curd and coconut paste and cook for 2 minutes.
- Add curry leaves and oil. Mix well and serve.

Variations: Use tamarind or unripe mango instead of curd. In some parts of Kerala, a piece of bitter gourd is also added. This lends a certain piquancy to the dish.

Warming Jujube Tea

Ingredients

5–6 dried jujubes
10 dried goji berries
½-inch grated ginger
Small piece of Ceylon cinnamon
Honey or jaggery (optional)

Method

- Wash the dried jujubes and goji berries thoroughly.
- Deseed the jujubes and roughly chop them up.
- In a saucepan, add double the water, so if it's a large mug of tea, add twice the amount. First bring it to a boil with all ingredients (except honey or jaggery),

then simmer till half the water evaporates. Strain thoroughly, pressing down in the strainer with a spoon so that all liquid is extracted from the jujubes and berries. Once it cools down a bit add honey or jaggery to taste.

JASMINE AND PARIJAT

There's nothing more synonymous with India than the sweet smell of jasmine. We have so many varieties of this beautiful flower, each with its unique scent. There is the beautiful madhumalti, with its heady fragrance and flowers that turn from white to red as they age. There is the tiny, star-like juhi, the gandhraj or gardenia, with its creamy fragrance, the ubiquitous chandni, which though doesn't have fragrance, is a beautiful-looking tree. What is so special about jasmine flowers is that they have both day and night varieties, for instance raat ki rani and madhumalti, which are most fragrant at night. And though all plants are sacred, as they're created by the divine, the jasmine sambac and parijat hold a special place in mythology.

Jasmine sambac, also known as Arabian jasmine, bela or mallika in Hindi, and Madurai malli for its association with this temple town, is one of India's most celebrated flowers. Its creamy, enveloping fragrance, which is most potent after dusk, makes it the subject of legends and folklore. It is associated with romance and is a symbol of everlasting beauty and love. It is considered sacred too. There are many divine associations where it is offered to Lord Shiva and Parvati at temples, such as the Meenakshi Temple in Madurai and Mallikarjuna Swamy Temple in Srisailam. It was mentioned in the Shiva Purana, which can be dated around tenth–eleventh century CE. It is also among the five fragrant flowers that adorn the arrow of Kama, the god love, with the other five flowers being from the mango and Ashoka trees, plus the blue and white lotus. It's only natural that a flower as pristine and fragrant as jasmine sambac has its presence in poetry. In one of the Sangam poems (written between 100 and 250 CE), there is one about a king who was so distraught after seeing the jasmine vine on the hard forest floor that he gifted it his chariot so that the creeper could wrap itself around it and grow magnificently.

The parijat tree is known for its small, orange-stemmed blooms that unfurl at night and fall from the tree as soon as sunlight hits them in the morning. For this reason, this tree is also known as the tree of sorrow, as it sheds the flowers like tears. The tree holds an exalted position in Indian mythology. In the legendary story of Samudra manthan, or churning of the ocean of milk, this tree was one of the treasures that came out of the ocean and was claimed by Indra, the Vedic deity of rain, to adorn his abode in heaven. In another mythological story, it was Lord Krishna who stole this tree for his wife Satyabhama, who was enchanted with the heady fragrance of the parijat flowers. In yet another story, Parijata was a princess who fell in love with the sun god. When the sun deserted her, the princess committed suicide. This tree grew from her ashes and is considered to be her incarnation. The wounds of love sometimes last forever. It is believed that this reincarnated tree cannot stand the sight of the sun and therefore blooms only at night and sheds her blossoms as tears in the morning when touched by the first rays of sunlight.

Interestingly, there is some confusion about why the baobab tree from Africa is also considered to be parijat. For instance, there is a baobab tree at the Kintoor village in the Barabanki district, Uttar Pradesh, that is worshipped as the parijat tree. In fact, the story behind this tree is that it grew out of the ashes of Queen Kunti, the mother of Pandavas, which dates it around the time of the Mahabharata, which was written around the third century BCE. There are many theories as to how the African baobab tree found its way to India. Some say it was brought here by Nubian mistresses of kings. Others say it was brought by travellers such as Ibn Battuta. But even though it may be synonymous, it isn't the parijat as the baobab doesn't flower around festival seasons as mentioned in the epics. Ultimately a name is just a label. Every tree should be considered sacred, as it feeds the soil, and is home to birds, insects, animals and microbes. It is only when we see all trees as worthy of worship will we think twice about mindlessly felling them—as is the unfortunate trend today.

The Science

The fragrance of all varieties of jasmine is arousing and awakening for the human brain. Just a whiff of this beautiful flower fills the mind with joy and its oil is indeed stimulating. In aromatherapy, jasmine is used to alleviate fear and depression because it helps uplift the mood and instill confidence. To investigate this effect, researchers enlisted forty volunteers and massaged jasmine oil on the abdomen of these subjects. Compared with placebo, it was found that jasmine significantly increased breathing rate, blood oxygen and skin temperature, which are considered to be indicative of arousal. Therefore, it can be concluded that the application of jasmine oil can help uplift the mind and increase alertness. Interestingly, it was also found that jasmine tea, on the other hand, had a more sedative effect on autonomic nerve activity at a very low intensity. This happens because of R-(-)- linalool, which is the main component of jasmine. It has a more relaxing effect. In another Taiwanese study, it was found that jasmine helped activate the parasympathetic nervous system, which helps the body relax after periods of stress and danger. This proves its potential as an adjunct therapy to keep the mind alert and nervous system balanced.

Parijat, or harshingar, is a night-blooming jasmine that also has an extremely stimulating fragrance. The therapeutic effects of its leaves are well known. In fact, its leaves were utilized in a decoction in India during the Covid pandemic. It has been found that the leaves of this plant do have antihistaminic, anti-inflammatory, antibacterial and anti-fungal activity. In a study, volunteers were given a paste of five freshly plucked parijat leaves which came to approximately 7 g per person. Their age range was 15–55 years and all of them were confirmed to have malaria. The doses were divided into one in the morning, then in the afternoon and the final installment at dinner, for a period of seven days, which led to parasitic clearance in the majority of the volunteers. While we do need more research to understand whether it can be used in medicine, there is no doubt that as an adjunct therapy, it can be utilized in decoctions, teas and as a part of green juices for its multitude of benefits.

Parijat Kadha

Ingredients

5 parijat leaves
3 tulsi leaves
1 clove
2 peppercorns
Small piece of Ceylon cinnamon

Method

- Grind the parijat and tulsi leaves to a rough paste.
- In a pan, boil all the ingredients in a large glass of water and continue boiling till the liquid evaporates to half its quantity.
- You may add 1 tsp of good-quality raw honey if you want to increase its antibacterial qualities. Drink this every day to soothe your throat and to boost immunity. It is also good for fever, respiratory allergies and cough.

Awakening Essential Oil Blend

Ingredients

2 drops of jasmine essential oil
4 drops of sandalwood essential oil
3 drops of palmarosa essential oil
2 drops of vanilla essential oil
30 ml almond oil

Method

Blend all of these together, shake well and let it rest for a day, before you begin using this essential oil blend to calm your mind, energize your senses and feel alert. To use this oil, take two drops, rub it between your palms and inhale deeply.

POMEGRANATE

There are some fruits that are considered blessed across all cultures; pomegranate is one of them. Whether as a symbol of abundance or purity, this nourishing fruit is ubiquitous around the world. In the Quran, it is mentioned three times. In fact, the Prophet himself has said that: 'There is no pomegranate unless there is a seed in it from paradise and I would like not to miss a single seed.' In Buddhism, it is considered one of the three sacred/blessed fruits, the others being peach and citrus. There is one particular story in which the demoness Hariti was cured of her taste of devouring children after she ate a pomegranate gifted by the Buddha. In China, Japan and Christian art, the pomegranate is seen as a symbol of fertility and abundance. Greek legends are, in fact, replete with mentions of the pomegranate fruit or tree, whether it is in the not-so-fortunate story of Goddess Persephone or the more optimistic symbolism in the story of Leucippe and Clitophon, where the two lovers give thanks for safe travels before the statue of Zeus, holding a pomegranate.

Historians have often wondered whether it was the date palm or pomegranate tree that was depicted as the tree of life in ancient paintings from the Mesopotamian civilization. A list of perfume ingredients from Pliny's ancient encyclopedia called *Natural History* included pomegranate rind and juice as materials for fragrance. Though it has been adopted by many cultures around the world, it is believed that it first grew in East Mesopotamia during the early Bronze Age and was well established by the middle Bronze age, having spread to countries such as Egypt, where it was not a native tree. The Egyptians depicted this tree in their murals, planted it in temples, used it to flavour wines, colour fabrics, in medicine and cosmetics. It was also used symbolically in funeral offerings as ivory and stone pomegranates. Plus, pomegranate-shaped golden pendants were found in Tutankhamun's tomb. Though the Egyptians did not consider it to be a sacred tree, it was nevertheless a symbol of fertility due to its multiple seeds.

In India, this fruit is offered to both Durga and Ganesha. In the Ganesha Bhujangam Stotra, a line in the verse describes Ganesha holding the beejapuram (another name for pomegranate because of its multiple seeds) in his trunk. Indeed, this fruit is revered and considered sacred all around the world and deservingly so, because from seed to skin, it has a multitude of benefits making it a wonderful addition to diet, nutraceuticals and cosmetics.

The Science

Pomegranate is revered for good reason, as it has one of the highest amounts of antioxidants. It also increases haemoglobin and is therefore useful in anaemia. If you were to choose one fruit, make it the pomegranate because of its vast benefits for health. This fruit is especially rich in ellagitannin, a type of tannin that is widely used in plastic surgeries due to its antioxidant effects that preserve skin health. The other antioxidants are anthocyanins, which are also found in blueberries, and the peel is high in catechins, which is also the active ingredient of green tea. Because of this the antioxidant potential of pomegranate is higher than that of green tea and red wine, both of which are considered as antioxidant superfoods. The seed contains punicic acid, which is its main constituent, and has been studied for its effect introducing the plaque within the arteries.

While fruit juices are mostly not recommended, since they contain high amounts of sugar, an exception can be made for pomegranate, as concentrated pomegranate juice was found to reduce heart disease risk factor and also helps in fatty liver disease. The peel of this fruit is more medicinal than the fruit itself and it has been proven that the dried powder of pomegranate peel helps inhibit candida infections. Because of this effect, it has been studied for dental potential where the pill showed strong effects against candida and had an anti-plaque effect when the peel powder was used as part of a mouth rinse.

Higher antioxidant content naturally translates into the fruit being excellent for skin health. Studies have shown that application and consumption of pomegranate helps guard the complexion against UV damage. Pomegranate seed oil is also excellent for the skin, as it helps thicken the density and improves firmness by stimulating the skin's production of collagen, elastin and hyaluronic acid. It also prevents the formation of new blood vessels, thereby reducing the appearance of redness. These benefits are because of the presence of punicic acid, which has potent anti-inflammatory, antibacterial and antioxidative effects, plus it helps reduce swelling in the tissues. This makes pomegranate the queen of fruits, which is beneficial whether it is eaten or applied.

Application

The easiest way to make pomegranates a part of your life is to eat one pomegranate every day. When I had several surgeries for endometriosis, eating one pomegranate every day was something my gynaecologist recommended, and I followed it religiously. But why eat only the fruit when the peel has even higher antioxidant capability? Pomegranate peel powder is easily available and can be stirred into smoothies or infused in herbal teas. Additionally, one can employ cold-pressed pomegranate seed oil for massage to strengthen and thicken the skin.

Liver-Friendly Red Juice

Ingredients

1 beetroot
1 red capsicum
10 curry leaves
½ pomegranate fruit
A strip of pomegranate peel (organic) or 1 tsp pomegranate peel powder

Method

Blend everything together. Then strain and drink the juice with a squeeze of lemon.

Infused Face Oil

Ingredients

20 ml cold-pressed pomegranate seed oil
10 ml cold-pressed almond oil

A chef's pinch of saffron
1 tbsp dried calendula flowers

Method

- Blend all the ingredients together in a glass jar.
- Keep this jar covered with the cloth in a sunny spot for 15 days to a month so that the herbs infuse into the oil.
- Then strain and use as an oil for face massage.

RICE AND BARLEY

Whether grains hold an exalted position in religions around the world isn't the point. The fact is that they are a source of sustenance and that itself makes them sacred. Food is divine and when we eat, we must do so with great reverence, as every morsel contains the heat from the sun, the moisture of the earth and the toil of the farmer. It's no surprise then that grains are deified in every culture. In the Vedas, rice is said to have been made from the mysterious heavenly drink soma. Later, in the Mahabharata, there was the story of Krishna, who visited the impoverished Draupadi and the Pandavas in the forest. All she had to offer him was a grain of rice, which magically multiplied in the earthen pot to feed not only Krishna but all the five Pandava brothers. The lesson was not to waste even a grain of rice. Indeed, the true worship of food grains is not to waste a single morsel.

In Buddhism, rice is venerated, as when Siddhartha Gautam was enlightened and became Gautama Buddha after a deep and lengthy meditation, it was a bowl of kheer, or rice pudding, that revived his health. In Indonesia, Dewi Sri, the rice goddess, is revered among farmers as someone who has the power to bestow a long life, fertility, wealth and children. Interestingly, Sri is another name for Goddess Lakshmi, who is also known as Annapurna, goddess of food and feeding. In Japan, rice is associated with the sun goddess Amaterasu, who is believed to have invented the cultivation of rice and wheat. Emperor Jimmu, the legendary first emperor of Japan, is the grandson of this sun goddess, who gives him the original rice grains that she had sown in heaven. The intention was to transform Japan from wilderness to a land of succulent rice nurtured by the sun goddess.

Rice is ubiquitous in customs, whether it's weddings or prayers. It is strewn on newlyweds to bless them with fertility and abundance. In Tripura, the tribes believe that drinking the locally brewed rice beer called chowak is representative of Goddess Lakshmi and is an essential part of all rituals from life to death, though its popularity is currently waning because of modernization and commercialization. On the other side of the world, in the United States, the indigenous people in the Great Lakes area consider Manoomin, the Ojibe word for wild rice that grows in the shallow areas of these lakes as sacred since it provides physical and spiritual sustenance. In India, a special kind of variety, native to

Kerala, known as Navara rice, is considered sacred and offered in temples. It is also extensively used in Ayurveda for consumption and application. To be used in therapies, this rice is cooked in a decoction of herbs and filled into poultices to be used in massage, which is very nourishing and gives strength to muscles and tendons.

Another grain that is sacred and ancient is barley. It is used in many rituals: during Navaratri (celebrating nine days of the goddess), in weddings and funerals. It is also an essential part of homa or havan. One of the qualities of barley is its ability to adapt to various climates— including the harsh environment of the Arctic Circle and Tibet—along with its short-growing period that makes it an excellent cash crop. The reverence of plants that provide us with food reaches its zenith among the Shuhi people—a Tibeto–Burman group of about 1500 people living in South-West Sichuan—who have a deep knowledge of and respect for plants. The Shuhi practise crop rotation, planting wheat and barley during winter, and maize and wet rice during summer. They spread organic fertilizer twice a year (manure mixed with oak leaves) and during Tibetan New Year in December, they sow a variety of plants between the wheat and barley to ask the gods for good growth and large yields. This offering, known as *telasyi*, consists of plants such as laato kath or oblong petal dogwood, a type of golden bamboo and Yunnan pine, among others. During spring, a similar ceremony is done for rice seedlings, where clematis and other flowering plants are offered, as rice is believed to be fond of flowers. Some may brush these rituals away as mere superstitions, however most of these rituals have a deeper meaning and wisdom. It is entirely possible that these plants that are offered to the gods for better yield could in fact be the perfect neighbour plants for the cash crops being grown. In any case, biodiversity, where multiple plants are being grown instead of monocultures that focus on a single crop, is infinitely better for soil quality, as it supports a variety of microorganisms that enrich the earth.

There are remains of barley grains found at archeological sites in fertile crescent in the Middle East that was home to some of the earliest civilizations, which indicates that the grain was domesticated around 10,000 years ago. Barley was also found to be one of the staple foods in the Indus Valley Civilization. Yava, which translates to barley corn, was a name for a unit of measurement (about one-third of an inch) in ancient India and it was also used as a unit of measurement in Tibet. Barley was mentioned in the Vedic and Tantric texts and continues to be revered as part of important events and celebrations today. This hardy grain hasn't just lasted through civilizations across the years but has also been continually worshipped.

The Science

Rice and barley are staple foods of people all over the world and have been consumed over the centuries. Recently though, there has been a push against carbohydrates in general. And because we are consuming so much of refined carbs, it is assumed that rice is nothing but sugar. The truth is, it is an important source of fibre, minerals, proteins, antioxidants and of course energy, which fuels us through the day. Think about it; peptides are extracted from rice, there are protein powders made from it, so to just view it as a source of pure carbs and nothing else is a great injustice to this wonderful grain. Rice is hypoallergenic in nature as compared to other grains such as wheat or even some millets, which perhaps don't suit everyone. According to Ayurveda, rice is extremely cooling and nourishing in nature; therefore, it is wonderful for people who have acneic skin and for all those who are prone to rosacea.

Whole grains form the backbone of diet in Blue Zones, where people tend to live until 100 years of age. Therefore, grains are most advantageous in their unrefined form when they are eaten whole with their bran. Brown rice, for instance, contains thiamine riboflavin, niacin, Vitamin E, iron, zinc, amino acids and more. The bran itself contains many advantageous components that are effective against diabetes and helps reduce cholesterol absorption. The good news is that rice comes in many varieties and colours, all with a different micronutrient profile. So just as we rotate different types of oils, vegetables, leafy greens and fruit in our diet, so should we try different varieties of rice. Different colours of rice indicate various levels of anthocyanins because of which we see colours such as brown, red, black and purple. Red rice is enriched with iron and zinc, whereas black rice contains protein fat and crude fibre. There are many varieties of rice, especially in south India, which are known for their medicinal properties. For instance, the kavuni has antimicrobial qualities, poongar is believed to enhance the reproductive health of women, kattu yanam lowers blood glucose levels and give strength, and mapiillai samba is supposed to enhance the fertility of men. Then of course there is the Navara red rice, which is extensively used in Ayurvedic therapies and face packs as well as for internal ailments such as stomach ulcers.

And then there's barley, which is valued not only for its grain but recently we have also seen a surge in the popularity of barley grass. Data supports the claim that barley grass is perhaps one of the most important functional foods that helps to prevent chronic disease, as it is rich in gamma-aminobutyric acid (GABA), flavonoids, superoxide dismutase, calcium, vitamins and tryptophan. It also contains one of the highest mineral content, especially potassium, calcium, iron and sulfur along with vitamins A, C, E and K. When we consume this grass daily, it helps us sleep better. It also reduces blood sugar and pressure, boosts immunity and liver function, detoxifies the body helping in acneic skin, prevents constipation, reduces inflammation, provides relief in dermatitis, reduces fatigue and improves memory. New research also indicates that it may have the ability to degrade six different types of pesticides.

I love barley because it's used for multiple purposes. It is used as green fodder for animals, the straw is used as animal bedding or for thatched roofs, as a grain, and of course, as we just discussed, it is a functional food. Barley grain contains the lowest Glycaemic Index (GI), and the most amount of beneficial beta glucans, resistant starch and antioxidant content of any cereal. Low GI means that the carbohydrates break down slowly and do not cause your blood sugar to spike. Resistant starch is like a probiotic for the good bacteria in your gut, whereas beta glucans are soluble fibres. Just like rice, barley also comes in red and purple varieties, though they are hard to find. They contain a different and higher antioxidant content than regular barley. However, unlike rice, barley is not gluten free. Therefore, this grain should be avoided by people who have celiac disease or gluten intolerance.

Pazhamkanji (Fermented Rice Gruel)

Ingredients

Leftover rice
Water
Shallots
Green chillies

Method

- Boil indigenous rice in an earthen pot (one part rice and three parts water).
- Once cooked, turn the stove off and let the mixture cool to lukewarm.
- Add a handful of pounded shallots and green chillies to the earthen pot of cooked rice and water.
- Leave the mixture overnight. An overnight fermentation bio-emboldens this mix with gut-friendly nutrients and minerals.
- Have the gruel as your first meal with a cup of fresh yogurt.

Rice Ferment for Hair

Ingredients

A fistful of white rice
Sufficient drinking water to soak and boil the rice

Method

This ferment can be made in two ways: either soak the rice and drain the water, which can be fermented, or boil the rice and instead of draining, use the water after boiling. I like to use both types of water. I ferment both separately in different glass bottles. To ferment this water, pour it into a glass jar or bottle, then use a square strip of cloth to cover the mouth of the bottle or the jar and secure it around the neck with a rubber band. Leave it to ferment for two days.

When the water is ready, you can use it in many ways: you can either use this as a last rinse after a shampoo, spray it all over your hair or massage it deep into the roots like a hair oil. I like to spray it all over my hair and massage it into my roots leaving it on for an hour before I rinse it out. Be warned that the water smells strongly and may not be suitable if you are sensitive to strong smells. This water helps soften the hair and may also help thicken your hair.

How to Grow Barley Grass

Ingredients

A cup of barley seeds
A shallow container or terracotta planter
Potting soil enriched with compost
A spray bottle

Method

Soak the barley grass in water overnight. In the morning, line the shallow container or planter with an inch or two of soil. Pour over the soaked barley seeds and spread them uniformly. Then cover with a thin layer of soil. Spray every day with water and watch the seeds grow into grass. Keep another container ready with soil to grow fresh seeds as grass grown a second or third time with the old seeds will lose its potency.

Navara Rice Face Mask

Ingredients

1 heaped tsp Navara rice powder
A splash of raw milk
½ tsp raw honey

Method

Mix all the ingredients to make a spreadable paste. Apply it on your face and neck and wash off after 20 minutes to soothe, comfort and hydrate your skin.

LOTUS AND HIBISCUS

The plants that are especially revered are worshipped for a reason. It could be for their nutritious qualities or the ability to protect the environment; it could be their history that goes back for millennia, or multiple uses of each and every part of the plant. With the sacred lotus flower, it is all of the above. Just like coconut, lotus too goes back millions of years, as scientists suggest it could even be 135 million years old, when it existed in the Northern Hemisphere and made its home in water. Unlike other plants that were destroyed in the Ice Age, lotus survived and is present and thriving even today. Its presence is interwoven into the fabric of our lives. It is worshipped in several religions and is a symbol of purity and durability.

The Hindi word for this flower is 'pankaja', which means one that grows in mud. Every evening, the flower submerges under shallow, muddy waters and rises each morning, pristine and gleaming. It is a proven fact that lotus seeds can survive for thousands of years as observed with a sacred lotus seed (*Nelumbo nucifera*) from China that germinated after 1300 years. In Hinduism, every variety of lotus is associated with a different god. The pink/red lotus is associated with Goddess Lakshmi and Lord Vishnu, the god who preserves all of creation. In one version of how the cosmos came into being, there is a story in the Vishnu Purana of how a lotus sprouting out of Vishnu's navel gave birth to the universe. The white lotus is associated with Brahma, who rules all of creation. And then there is the blue lotus, which technically is a water lily, but is associated with Shiva, the god of destruction.

In ancient Egypt, the lotus takes on a more phallic significance, as it is associated with the sun, life, immortality and resurrection since it reappears from murky waters every morning. In some artefacts, Ra, the Egyptian sun god, is depicted as a child who sleeps on a lotus. Incidentally, Lord Surya, the sun god, also holds a lotus in his hand. In tantra, the lotus is a part of the yantras, or diagrams that symbolize the womb and womanhood. Buddhists see the flower as a symbol of enlightenment for the same quality—the ability to rise above the murk and chaos of everyday life. In fact, the Buddhist mantra 'om mani padme hum', when translated means the jewel in the lotus, which represents awakening and transcendence. Interestingly, in Ayurveda, it is said that the heart is in the shape of an inverted lotus.

Typically, red flowers are offered to goddesses and white flowers to gods. For instance, jasmine is Krishna's favourite and white lotus is for Brahma. On the other hand, red lotus is for Goddess Lakshmi.

The other flower that is popular as an offering to goddesses is red hibiscus, which is offered to Goddess Kali. The bright-red petal of the hibiscus is supposed to be symbolic of the red tongue of Kali and is ubiquitous in the goddesses' temples, especially in Bengal. It is believed that it can eliminate negative energy in the place that it is planted in just like the goddesses that is related to it, i.e. Kali and Durga. Throughout history, it has been employed in cosmetics and medicine from the Caribbean to India and China. It is an ornamental plant, but it's not merely beautiful. It also plays a significant role in medicine, cosmetics, nutrition and the environment.

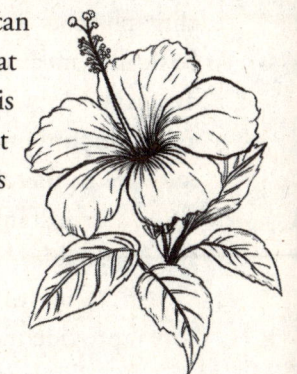

The Science

Though the lotus is seen as the ceremonial flower of ancient origin, it is a symbol of evolutionary sophistication that has adapted over millennia to what we see it as today. This remarkable plant can withstand environmental stressors because of its seeds, which have the ability to remain dormant for centuries and which contribute to its survival. Additionally, the leaves have a unique hydrophobic ability to repel water-based sediments and remain clean. The flower has an interesting self-heating mechanism which ensures that it stays within the range of a comfortable 30–36°C even though the surrounding temperatures may fluctuate between 10 and 45°C.

The lotus plant is truly a symbol of purity, as it works like a biofilter in water bodies. It helps assimilate pollutants such as heavy metals and helps maintain nitrogen levels. Its wide saucer-shaped leaves and root system also provide shelter and food to a wide range of aquatic life. Moreover, this plant is excellent for carbon sequestration, which basically means the process of capturing and storing atmospheric carbon dioxide, making it an important tool for ecological purposes. Lotus plants can be harvested again and again; therefore, they are a great renewable source for fibre. For instance, lotus silk is a textile that is completely biodegradable.

In terms of food, both the seeds and roots of the lotus provide nourishment to humans. Lotus seeds are colloquially known as makhana, or fox nuts, though makhana is extracted not from lotus but from a species of waterlily that looks very similar to lotus. The local name for lotus seeds is 'kamal ka gatta'. These seeds are very nutritious and considered to be a complete source of plant-based protein, with all the amino acids, which is a rarity in vegetarian sources of protein. Though they are usually used in traditional customs, they can be added to soups and desserts too. Lotus root is commonly eaten in India as a side vegetable. It is extremely beneficial, as it is high in Vitamin C, calcium and fibre content. All in all, this plant provides sustenance to a variety of species and is important for ecological purposes too.

Just like the lotus works as an unnatural filter for water bodies, the ornamental hibiscus tree has the potential to clear heavy metals from the soil. Additionally, their brightly coloured flowers attract pollinators such as bees, butterflies and hummingbirds that form the backbone of our ecosystem. These flowers have been used extensively in haircare and even today the dried powder of these flowers can be used as a mild shampoo, perhaps because it is anti-fungal in nature, and it benefits the scalp. Though this plant comes in a variety of coloured blooms, the red-flowered variant is the one that is used in beauty preparations. Even when it is extremely popular in herbal preparations, there is little research done to back its usage in hair oils and hair packs. However, according to one study, an extract of hibiscus did have some hair growth-promoting properties. It has been revealed that it has anti-microbial and antioxidant properties, which also supports its traditional usage.

This plant is also extremely hardy, as it is resistant to pests, diseases, drought and waterlogging. It has a strong root system and survives in full sun, high heat as well as cold temperatures. While many consider this plant to be the source of the ever-popular, red-coloured hibiscus tea, the truth is that hibiscus tea is made from another species of this plant called roselle.

Application

These plants have woven themselves to the fabric of everyday Indian life. Hibiscus, of course, is easier to use because it is commonly planted in Indian homes. The flowers are used during pujas and are often added to hair oil, which interestingly gives it a blue tint. Many people like to grow lotus, especially if they have the space for a small pond in their homes. Lotus root, on the other hand, is fairly common and makes its appearance in many local dishes because of its versatility and delicious flavour.

Lotus Root Chips

Ingredients

2 thinly sliced lotus roots
Sendha namak/Himalayan pink salt to taste
1 tsp jeera powder
1 tsp red chilli powder
1 tbsp Samak rice powder
1 tsp oil
1 tsp honey

Method

- Peel and slice the lotus roots. Blanch them in hot salted water for 2 minutes.
- Blend Samak rice in a grinder to form a fine powder. Place sliced lotus stems in a bowl and add all the masalas and Samak rice powder, give it a nice toss making sure they are covered properly. Brush them with a little oil.
- Air fry them for 10–12 minutes. You can also add a bit of chaat masala if you wish.

Hibiscus Hair Oil

Ingredients

10 red hibiscus flowers
10 hibiscus leaves
1 tbsp fenugreek seeds
10–12 neem leaves
100 ml coconut oil

Method

- Heat the oil and add all the ingredients.
- Simmer on a low flame for about half an hour. Then cool and transfer into a glass jar.
- You may strain the mixture (though I like to retain all the ingredients in the oil).

SESAME, TURMERIC AND MUSTARD

Every year, in mid-January, North India celebrates Makar Sankranti, which marks the end of the harsh winter. During this festival, eating and donating sesame seeds as also bathing in its oil is considered to be auspicious. A day before this festival, Lohri is celebrated in Punjab, with sesame seeds-laced sweets offered to a raging bonfire. Both festivals celebrate the end of winter and the sowing season, with sesame seeds being the ideal seed for the sun god. Sesame has long been considered sacred. In the Atharva Veda, it is mentioned that the seed was never up for sale and was reserved for rituals only. Since then, it has many sacred associations, whether its association with Surya, the sun god, or Yama, the god of death, which makes this seed both a symbol of prosperity and immortality. Though both varieties of sesame are considered to be auspicious, the black sesame seeds are donated in the homa or havan. In the northern parts of India, where it grows plentifully, sesame seeds are ubiquitous in ceremonies, be it at weddings or funeral rites.

Though it is a seed, sesame (til) was considered as a cereal in the Harappan civilization, almost 3500 years ago. India was the birthplace of sesame and from here it moved towards Mesopotamia and China and is now cultivated all over the world. With the seeds travelled its sacred lore. Sesame was considered fit for kings and was found in the tomb of King Tutankhamen of Egypt, along with food, drinks, perfumes, ointments and oils. In Armenia, where sesame was seen as a symbol of beauty, it replaced olive oil in the anointing mixture and attracted criticism from the Greek orthodox church. In fact, the word 'til', which is what sesame is called in India, means 'to anoint'.

Though its uses were mostly sacred, a decoction of sesame seed mixed with linseed was used as an aphrodisiac in India and the Middle East. In the *Kama Sutra*, there is a recipe in which the covering of the sesame seed, when soaked in sparrow's eggs and boiled in milk, sugar and ghee, helped a man enjoy innumerable women. In the *Book of Cleopatra*, it was recommended to treat impotence, and the Sultan of Yemen suggested that sesame fried and eaten with hemp seeds increases desire. In fact, there were many preparations of sesame mixed with cannabis, one in particular in Egypt where wafers of sesame were pressed together with honey and interlaced with small particles of hashish. Not to mention the symbolism of sesame with familiar phrases such as 'open sesame' from the *Arabian Nights*, inspired by the seed's ability to split into two, plus its uses in occult and divination, which makes it one of the oldest and most revered seeds in the world.

But nothing is more symbolic of India as turmeric. This spice enjoys an exalted space not only in sacred rituals but also in celebrations, funerals, cosmetics, cuisine and even occult practices. It's been mentioned in the Vedas and has several mythological stories attached to it, most notably the story where Goddess Parvati would cleanse herself with turmeric paste and also created Lord Ganesha out of the paste. Other stories allude to its position as an offering to the sun god or symbolic of Goddess Durga, who is supposed to preside over this plant. Brides apply turmeric for weeks before their wedding, as it ensures clear and glowing skin. Some varieties of this spice are used on babies. It is also used to disinfect a house and is an integral part of various cuisines—all for its immunity-boosting, protective, antibacterial qualities. Naturally, it has stood the test of time and today not only is it interwoven in the fabric of daily life in India but is also a prime ingredient as an addition to cosmetic formulas or nutraceuticals.

The third herb ingredient that has powerful spiritual associations is the mustard tree. The parable of the mustard seed goes like this: 'The kingdom of heaven is like a mustard seed that someone took and sowed in his field; it is the smallest of all the seeds, but when it has grown, it is the greatest of shrubs and becomes a tree, so that the birds of the air come and make nests in its branches.' It basically means that even faith as small as a mustard seed is capable of moving mountains. The seed is also mentioned twice in the Quran, with hadiths or inspiring and poetic reminders of how the small size of the mustard has the potential to grow into a large, valuable plant. It is revered across cultures, whether it's in the West, the Middle East or India, where it is considered a symbol of protection and good luck.

The Science

These three ingredients, especially sesame and turmeric, are quite common in Indian cuisine. Mustard hasn't gained the popularity it so deserves. Its sharp flavour reflects its potent phytochemical make-up. Did you know that even broccoli belongs to Brassicaceae, the mustard family of flowering plants, with its trademark flavour, which perhaps is a sign of sinigrin, a compound associated with the mustard family? It has been found that Indian mustard (leaves and seeds) contains significant amounts of this compound, perhaps the highest in any sort of plant food. It was found that when sinigrin is metabolized by the body, it leads to the formation of other compounds called isothiocyanates, which contribute to antitumour activity, reduce triglycerides, and are praised for their anti-inflammatory and antioxidant activity. Mustard cake is also used as a biofertilizer because of the presence of glucosinolates, such as sinigrin, which help control as well as boost plant growth.

Though mustard oil contains low saturated fat, it is a rich source of glucosinolates and omega-3 fatty acids. Internationally, there is still hesitancy towards its consumption because of high levels of erucic acid, which has been found to cause heart problems in animal studies. In India, we tend to almost burn the mustard oil till it forms a plume of smoke. Perhaps that is to eliminate this erucic acid. However, more studies are required to understand this mechanism. Personally, I love cooking my greens in cold-pressed mustard oil. In fact, eggs taste surprisingly good when cooked in this pungent-tasting oil.

Another seed that is prized for its oil is sesame, which has the highest oil content among all oil-producing crops—about 45–75 per cent, thus earning the moniker 'queen of oil'. It has a balanced omega-3 six and nine ratio and contains about twelve unsaturated fatty acids. Sesame is also one of those rare plant foods that can be considered a complete protein because it contains all the amino acids. In fact, even sesame oil meal contains about 50 per cent protein, while black sesame has more protein than the other varieties.

The highlight of sesame are the lignans, which are strong antioxidants that help regulate blood lipids and improve liver function. Again, the lignan content of black sesame seeds is higher than the other varieties. There are twenty-six lignans in sesame seeds and among these the most important is sesamin, a great antioxidant that helps lower cholesterol, stabilize blood pressure and metabolize lipids. It has also been found that sesame oil has anti-inflammatory, emollient effects and it also helps reduce swelling. Perhaps this is why it is used extensively for massage and oil pulling in Ayurveda. Whole sesame seeds with skin also work wonders as probiotics, i.e., food for gut bacteria. All in all, sesame is a highly versatile plant and can be used for various purposes.

The one spice that has been consistently related to good health and Indian practices is of course turmeric, which is now immensely popular all over the world, especially because curcumin, its active ingredient, has proved to be beneficial in health and beauty. But turmeric is so much more than just curcumin. Its fragrance comes from bioactives known as turmerones; in fact, it was found that turmerones are at par with curcuminoids and when combined together, their effect was even more robust. These turmerones are being studied to understand how they affect conditions such as cancer and Parkinson's disease. This proves that the benefits of whole turmeric are undeniable, and it is unfair to simply focus on curcumin. Because of its neuroprotective effects, turmeric helps boost brain health. Additionally, it is a powerful antioxidant, helps reduce inflammation, protects the heart and liver, has antiviral, anti-fungal and antibacterial effects, and detoxifies the body.

The only downside to turmeric is that because of its popularity, much of the turmeric powder we find in markets today is adulterated. Therefore, it is ideal to either choose a trustworthy organic brand or get dry turmeric roots that you get ground into powder in the market. You can mix it into a curry, which is its ideal medium, as curry contains other spices and fats that help turmeric get absorbed into the body. In winter, you can add it to your milk with a pinch of pepper. You can also add fresh turmeric juice to your winter smoothie or green juice.

There is an Ayurvedic combination known as haridrakumari, which combines turmeric with aloe vera. It is excellent for liver health, functions as a blood purifier and is used to treat skin disorders such as fungal infections and psoriasis. It is important to note however that turmeric can be heating in nature and should only be eaten as a part of curries in summer.

Application

These three ingredients are already part of our everyday lives. Turmeric and mustard seeds are regularly used in curries, but the usage of sesame is limited to winter and with good reason because these seeds are warming in nature. During the cold season, there are many sesame seed preparations such as ladoos and sesame candies, however they can be added to smoothies or sprinkled on top of breakfast cereals to ensure you get all the benefits of sesame seeds but without the added refined sugar.

Sesame and Roasted Besan Ladoos/Energy Balls

Ingredients

100 g white sesame
100 g besan (gram flour)
20 g fresh coconut (grated)
5 g/1 tsp cardamom powder
70 g jaggery/gud
20 g ghee
15 g pista
A pinch of salt

Method

- Roast the sesame in a pan till slightly brown. It is normal to hear a popping sound. Don't roast them too much. They tend to turn black and taste bitter. Remove from the pan and transfer to a plate immediately.
- Roast the besan till brown and keep aside.
- Roast the freshly grated coconut in a pan till brown and keep aside.
- Roast the pista and set aside.
- Transfer the roasted sesame, besan, pista and coconut to a mixee.
- Add the jaggery, cardamom powder and salt to the mix.
- Blend the mixer till it's semi-fine. Make sure you don't over blend it, otherwise it will turn wet and start to form a thick paste.
- Tranfer to a bowl.
- Add the ghee and mix it with your hand or a spoon.
- Make small balls and refrigerate for 30 minutes.

Golden Milk

Ingredients

A cup of milk (or nut milk)
¼ tsp of Lakadong turmeric or any other good-quality turmeric
A pinch of Ceylon cinnamon powder
3 threads of saffron

Method

- Mix all the ingredients together except the saffron.
- First, quickly bring them to a boil and then simmer for a few minutes.
- Once you take the milk off the heat and pour into a cup, add the saffron and mix into the milk. It is best enjoyed during winter.

Mustard Fertilizer

Ingredients

1 kg of mustard cake (mustard khali)
½ bucket of water

Method

Soak the mustard seed cake in water and keep it covered for about two weeks so that the water ferments. Add more water to the mixture and use it to water especially flowering plants.

APARAJITA AND CROWN FLOWER

Among the flowers offered to the gods and goddesses, there are some that are cultivated and others that grow on wastelands. For instance, the cultivated blue aparajita flower and the crown flower, which grows in wastelands. Both are revered and yet both grow in very different conditions. This contrast is important to illustrate because sometimes I find gardeners eschewing the common varieties of plants for the more exotic and expensive ones. When both flowers are fit for worship, who are we to differentiate?

Crown flower, also known as aak and madar, is a flower used to worship Shiva and Ganesha. It is believed that planting this shrub on the periphery or entrance of a house protects it from negative energy and helps eliminate evil eye directed to the members of the house. Though beliefs such as these are not rooted in science, I like to mention them, so that we can begin looking at trees and shrubs as sacred and divine creatures. The flowers are used in prayers and magical tantric ceremonies. Interestingly, they are also known as courage flowers, perhaps because they have the ability to grow in wastelands. Additionally, this plant has a variety of uses, for instance, it was used to makes textiles in Cyprus in 2000 BCE, charcoal from the wood was used in gun powder and fireworks in Indo-China, and the latex of these plants was used as an arrow poison in Africa. But from the most potent poisons come effective medicines. Therefore, this plant was treasured not only in the Ayurvedic materia medica but is also currently showing promise in its uses as a fungicide, insecticide, pesticide and as a bio-remediator.

Another blue-tinted flowering plant that is revered in both mythology and Ayurveda is the blue butterfly pea plant, also known as aparajita or the undefeated one. Considered to be an offering for Goddess Durga and gods Shiva and Shani, this is also prized for its brain-boosting ability. Its conch-shaped flowers have some physicians identify this plant as shankhapushpi from ancient texts, which isn't accurate. Still, like the shankhapushpi, this plant too has conch-shaped flowers that are associated with its balancing effect on the brain, which make this plant valuable for its nutritional and medicinal application.

The Science

It has always been valued in Ayurveda as a memory enhancer, as a sedative and for its anti-stress effects. In recent times, the aparajita plant has garnered a lot of attention for its application in farming and medicine. It is used in farming, as it has the ability to suppress weeds and enrich the soil by balancing the nitrogen content. Additionally, it's also a source of fodder for the cattle and can be used as green manure. The flower contains both alkaloids and glycosides; alkaloids help calm the nervous system, while glucosides are known for their anti-inflammatory and antioxidant properties. The extracts from this plant have shown to have antimicrobial, antiparasitic, antioxidant and neuroprotective qualities. Animal studies have shown that the extracts also have potential antidiabetic effects, while extracts from the seed and roots have shown remarkable wound-healing abilities.

While the aparajita flower has been used commonly to make teas and sherberts, the crown flower is extremely toxic to humans because of compounds known as phorbol esters, which are found in its milky sap. But it is common knowledge that the most potent medicine is made from the deadliest poisons. Still, it is imperative that the crown flower should not be used directly and kept away from children and animals. After being distilled, it is used as a medicine, be it in traditional or contemporary practices. Therefore, it's not surprising that it is used against diarrhoea and candida because of its potent antibacterial, antimicrobial and wound-healing ability.

Application

The best way to use crown flowers is to plant them around your house, as the flowers are a huge attraction for pollinators, such as butterflies. It is also a drought-resistant plant that requires very little care. Of course, traditionally, it's been used for centuries as a totem to ward off negativity and evil around the house. The best way to use aparajita is to infuse it in tea. You can either use fresh blooms or buy a packet of dried-up flowers that are easily available. This plant too is a huge attraction for pollinators and is wonderful to grow even in a large pot.

'Itminan' Tisane

Ingredients

1 tsp dried aparajita flowers
½ tsp dried chamomile flowers
¼ tsp dried lavender flowers
A small piece of fresh ginger (about ¼ inch), thinly sliced
1 cup hot water
Honey to taste (optional)

Method

- Combine the aparajita flowers, chamomile, lavender and ginger in a tea infuser or directly in a cup.
- Pour hot water (around 95 degree Celsius) over the bouquet.
- Steep for 5 minutes and strain the tisane.
- Sip Itminan by yourself or with your loved ones.

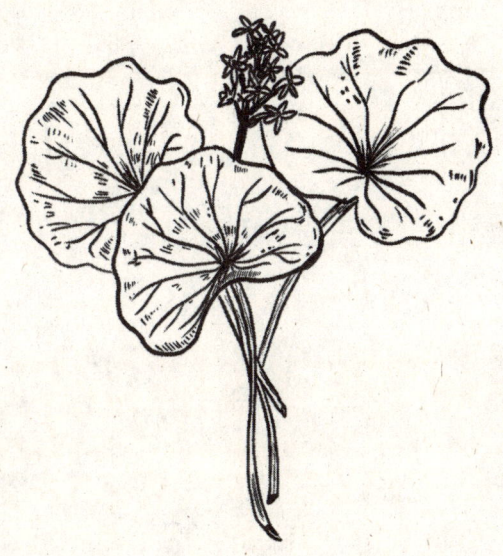

PART III

Sanctify

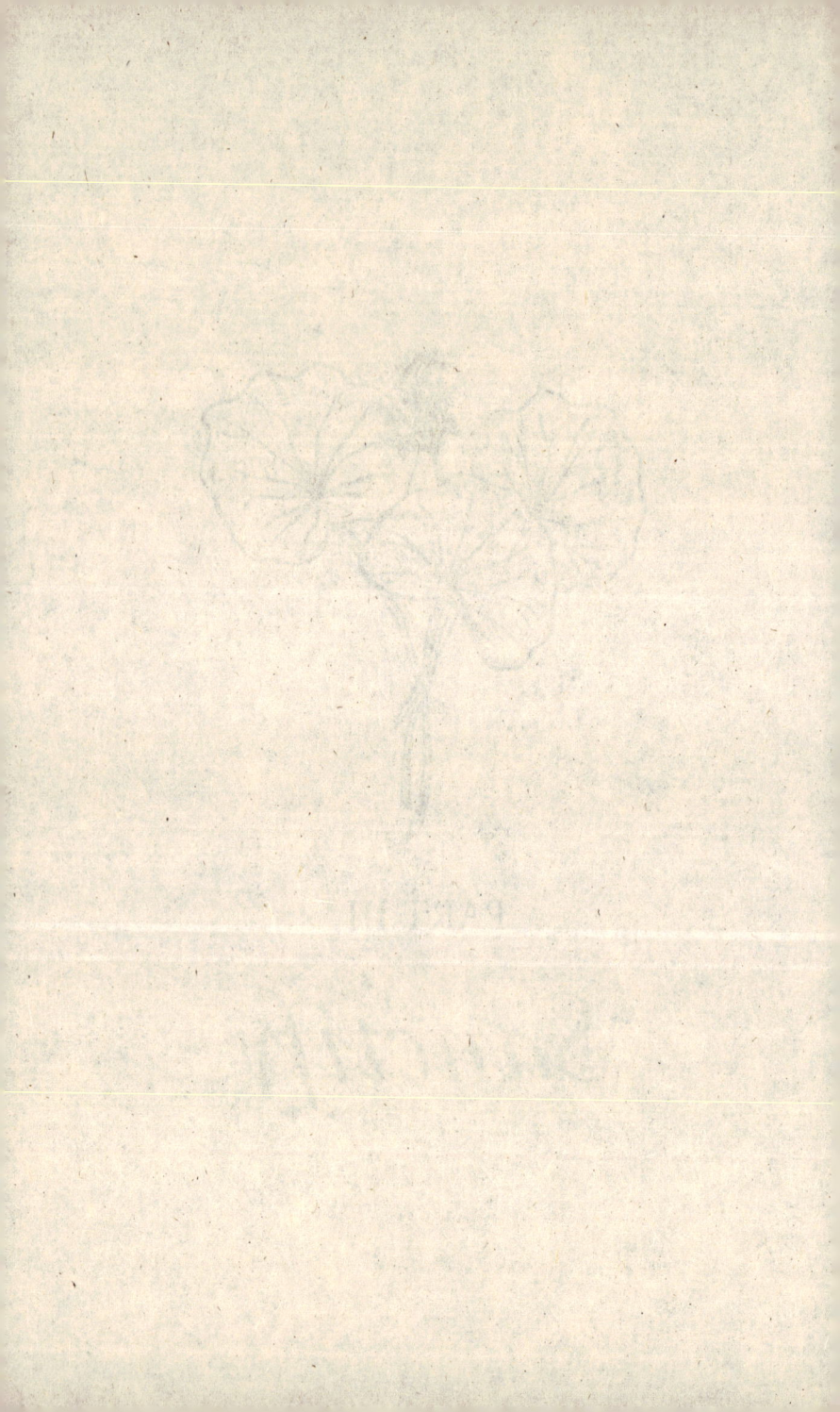

INTRODUCTION

The meaning of 'sanctify' is to make something pure or holy. But how do we define purity or holiness? Not by the narrow lens that leads to hate and acts of degradation against others. The perceived image of impurity has led to grave injustice against women and the weaker sections of society. Religion, personal choices or gender doesn't determine purity. After all, who are we to determine what is right or wrong? However, it is undeniable that being in the lap of nature feels purifying, and almost spiritual. Therefore, it is not surprising that we deem certain trees as holy and use their leaves to sanctify our homes and in places of worship.

The germ of an idea for this book arose from the legendary peepal. In India, we have all grown up with myths surrounding this majestic tree—from gods and goddesses living within its leaves and branches to it being haunted. Last year, when I wanted to plant one in our community garden, I came across another myth—that even the shadow of the peepal mustn't fall on your house, or it will attract great misfortune, which is why it must only be planted close to temples and never one's home. This led me down a rabbit hole to research what is it about this tree that makes it so intimidating. The answer lies in its wide and invasive root system, which can destroy the foundation of a house. Therefore, it is correct that it shouldn't be planted close to homes—but that's because of its widespread root system and not because it is inauspicious.

India considers most of its trees as sacred. Most are medicinal and provide great benefits to the air and soil quality. But several are enmeshed in superstition, like the tamarind tree, which is supposedly the abode of witches. The problem with this sort of folklore is that it prevents us from planting these trees that provide great environmental benefits. For instance, the banyan tree is also supposed to be a dwelling place for ghosts. However, the banyan is such a majestic tree that it supports an entire ecosystem consisting of various mammals, pollinators, microbes and even human beings who find shelter under its wide canopy.

For me, every plant, tree and herb is sacred because it is a creation of the divine force. We have enough studies to prove that green cover makes us feel more relaxed and concrete makes us feel more anxious. For me, anything natural takes us closer to the source. Therefore, one must see the divinity in every blade of grass and respect it as such. And every type of tree shows us a different face of the divine energy and its creativity in crafting so many different types of leaves, trunks, fruit, flowers, branches and canopies. Therefore, we must sanctify our gardens and homes with several varieties of plants not only for biodiversity that supports a wide variety of pollinators and microbes but also as a nod to the diversity provided to us by the earth goddess herself.

RUDRAKSHA AND TULSI

Mythology and folklore are replete with hundreds of tales according to which flowers, fruits, trees and shrubs are the abode of the divine. Among these, the king and queen of Indian herbs—rudraksha and tulsi—stand out with their exalted status in prayer and worship. Rudraksha has mystical associations. The name literally translates as 'tears of Rudra'—'Rudra' being the earliest name of Shiva. There are many tales about why he shed these tears. According to the Shiva Purana, the tree was born out of the tears of rage Lord Shiva shed when he destroyed the demon Tripurasura. Another story says that it was the sweat from his forehead while in deep meditation that fell to the ground and gave birth to this magnificent tree. Yet another legend goes that when he opened his eyes after thousands of years in meditation, tears filled his eyes out of deep compassion. And then there's the story of his grief on losing his wife, Sati, that caused tears to fall on earth giving birth to the rudraksha tree.

Because of its strong association with Shiva, this tree is considered to be the connection between heaven and earth. In fact, it is said that this sacred tree contains the secrets of the evolution of the cosmos within itself. It is believed that the bead has electromagnetic powers, which is why it is worn by mystics. According to Ayurveda, these beads help balance the heart and the nervous system. The quality of these beads are decided according to the number or lines of facets on them, which are known as *mukhi*s. For instance, a one-faced, or ek-mukhi, rudraksha is half-moon in shape and is associated with Shiva and enlightenment. On the other hand, a nine-faced, or nau-mukhi, rudraksha is associated with Goddess Durga and with living life fearlessly. The most commonly found type of bead is the five-faced, or paanch-mukhi, rudraksha and is associated with good health, peace and memory.

Rudraksha, though sacred, is used more by mystics as a protective amulet or in worship. Tulsi, the queen of herbs, however has woven itself into the fabric of Indian domesticity. Most homes have a tulsi plant: some worship it, while others consider it to be a lucky charm and hence keep it at the entrance of their home. Tulsi leaves can also be used as a superfood or to flavour salads and tea. Known as 'the incomparable one', this shrub was first mentioned in the Rig Veda and has been revered since. The story of its origin has several versions, but in a nutshell, this plant is a manifestation of Goddess Lakshmi, who is also the consort of Vishnu. Not only the shrub, even the soil around it is considered sacred. It is also believed that this plant purifies the aura of the house and keeping it with you is a connection with the divine. Of course, now we have scientific proof that tulsi has the power to protect tissues and organs against chemical stress, for instance, industrial pollutants and heavy metals as well as physical and mental stress. This goes to show that most rituals existed for a purpose and the worship and respect of plants is a mindset that must be cultivated in today's age, where we are losing our connection with nature. It's only when trees and plants are seen as divine that we will work to preserve nature and have any hopes of reversing the environmental damage that is now changing the world.

The Science

Both tulsi and rudraksha have been studied, however the former has more robust research behind it. That is not to say that the rudraksha has not been studied at all. There needs to be more research done, especially on the claims of rudraksha calming and stabilizing the human body because of its interaction with electromagnetic fields around us. Small studies, especially with plants, have found this claim to be somewhat true. It was found that in dhatura and vinca plants, the rudraksha bead stabilized flocculating current, which means energy in small clumps or masses, in these plants. In another study, where teen-mukhi, char-mukhi and paanch-mukhi rudraksha beads were ground and studied, it was found that they possess magnetic properties. In a small study conducted on ten people, it was found that these beads may improve oxygen levels and reduce pulse rates. However, a controlled clinical study or several studies are required to conclude for sure the scientific benefits of the rudraksha beads. Nonetheless, these small studies provide a sliver of evidence that these beads may indeed be beneficial.

A single tree contains all types of facets, or mukhis, from which beads can be made. Since it is pollinated by insects, the tree supports a large variety of pollinators, thereby making it excellent for the environment. It must be mentioned here however that this tree is difficult to grow, as it germinates very slowly from its seed. In fact, it takes about a year for the seed to sprout depending on the humidity of the soil. Additionally, the collection of seeds to make rosaries and beads impedes the natural regeneration of the rudraksha. Effort must be taken to ensure its numbers do not dwindle and that it does not go towards extinction. However, its growth and spread are already endangered because of the rampant seed collection and destruction of its natural habitats. While India is the largest consumer of rudraksha beads, it is also the largest importer of these beads, as it is an endangered tree. But if this tree is protected and grown as a source of income for the local population, perhaps there is a chance for it to grow and multiply reversing its endangered status.

On the other end of the spectrum is the tulsi plant. We have strong evidence to back its efficacy. It is grown in almost every home and is thereby not endangered at all. It is rightly known as the queen of herbs because it is the most effective adaptogen, meaning that it helps us cope very well with stress. One expert called it yoga for the mind. I love this description of tulsi because it does help the mind relax and makes it more alert at the same time, unlike caffeine, which makes us alert but also jittery. A cup of tulsi tea is my companion whenever I sit down to write. It enhances my focus and reduces stress. Tulsi is also the most researched as a radio-protective agent and helps protect us from pollution. Perhaps this is the reason why we have the tradition of planting tulsi in our homes.

But that's not all: tulsi has been found to be beneficial for several lifestyle-related disorders. One controlled trial found that consuming 2 g of powdered tulsi leaves, either alone or combined with curry leaves, led to a significant improvement in blood sugar levels after just two weeks. In another twelve-week randomized trial, it was found that 2 g of tulsi leaf extract, alone or combined with neem leaf extract, showed marked reduction in diabetic symptoms, with better effect shown with the combination of tulsi and neem. There is evidence to show significant improvement in blood pressure in hypertensive patients who were given 30 ml of fresh tulsi juice once or twice a day for 10–12 days. It was also found that there was an improvement in serum lipids in healthy adults who were given 300 mg of tulsi extract for four weeks and there was an improvement in lipid profile and BMI of obese participants who were given 250 mg capsules of this extract twice daily for eight weeks.

Tulsi is known to be excellent for asthmatic patients. 500 mg of dried leaves taken twice a day improves vital capacity, which is the capacity for amount of air a person can exhale after a maximum inhalation, and relief of asthmatic symptoms within three days, which shows that it can be used as an adjunctive therapy. This wonderful herb has also showed a positive effect on mood as demonstrated in three studies, with two studies reporting reductions of 31–39 per cent in overall stress-related symptoms in patients who have psychosomatic problems. Of course, this is not to say that tulsi should be seen as a replacement for medicines or drugs given to you by the doctor, but it definitely can be utilized as a lifestyle addition.

Let's not forget that even the seeds of tulsi (sabja), with its density of proteins, vitamins and minerals, are valued nutritionally. 100 g of sabja contains 11–22 per cent protein, dietary fibre between 7 and 26 g, and high amounts of minerals such as calcium, potassium and magnesium. Sabja is often confused with chia, but sabja is more cooling in nature. In fact, you may want to use this in place of chia seeds in the recipe for chia seed pudding during summer.

Application

Because of their spiritual associations, rudraksha beads are in high demand and naturally there are a lot of synthetic beads sold as the real thing. To test these for authenticity, one can place a bead between two copper coins. If it rotates slightly—indicating its electromagnetic effect—it is the real thing. Also, if you put the bead in the water, the real one will sink, whereas the synthetic version will float. Lastly, for rare beads such as Gauri Shankar Rudraksha and Tribhagi or Trijuti, where more than one bead is enjoined, one can boil them in water. If they are stuck with glue, the joint will change colour or fall apart.

If one needs to make rudraksha beads a part of their life, it is essential to find a trustworthy seller. The Nepalese rudraksha beads are considered to be the most powerful because of the pristine atmosphere they grow in. Just like other popular plant-based products, rudraksha too can be faked. Therefore, more than anything, it is essential to find a trustworthy seller and only wear the bead if it is prescribed to you rather than choosing one and wearing it on your own.

Tulsi, on the other hand, seamlessly blends into our everyday life. Swallow a tulsi leaf every morning with a glass of warm water to boost immunity and reduce inflammation because of its strong antioxidant profile. You can also make a paste of tulsi, amla and ginger to consume in the morning. I like to drink two–three cups of tulsi tea during the day while I work. To brew this tea, you just need to pour freshly boiled water over dried tulsi leaves and let it brew for a few minutes.

Immunity-Boosting Tulsi Paste

Ingredients

3–5 tulsi leaves
Half an amla
Half-inch ginger

Method

Make a shot with a little water and drink. Do not strain. You may also make a paste and consume it with warm water. This is a great shot for those living in a polluted environment. You may also grind all three into a paste and consume with it warm water in the morning. This paste is best consumed for 2–3 months in winter or around spring, not all through the year. Tulsi is best consumed as herbal tea during summer.

DURVA GRASS AND ARJUNA

The tale behind durva grass is a beautiful one and highlights its ability to reduce inflammation. As the story goes, this grass was offered to Lord Ganesha to calm down burning sensations. In one version, he is cursed by a celestial singer for spurning her marriage proposal and feels a burning sensation on his head, which calms down after he places a few blades of grass on his head. In another version, Ganesha swallows a demon who was destroying the world and after doing so he felt a burning sensation in his belly. Twenty-one stacks of this grass were offered by the rishis, which, upon consumption, calmed this sensation. Then there is the story that this grass became sacred when the drops of heavenly nectar fell upon it after the Samudra Manthan, or the divine churning of the ocean of milk by gods and demons.

The name durva is basically two words—*duhu* and *avam*—enmeshed together, which mean near and far. The word 'durva' is representative of the belief that this grass helps bring distant energy of the divine closer to the follower, with its three blades, which represent Ganesha and his parents, Shiva and Parvati. Despite its exalted status, the grass is generous in its growth and ubiquitous in grasslands and riversides. Interestingly, there are some parallels between the Indian worship of durva grass and the Native American reverence of sweet grass. According to one legend, sweet grass was used to transform a youth from the Piegan tribe (who was known as Scarface) into an attractive young man. Since then, twenty-one strands of sweet grass braided into one has become a sacred offering, similar to the twenty-one stacks of durva offered to Ganesha. In the Native American tradition, in the twenty-one blades, seven stand for the seven generations that came before, the next seven for seven teachings of love, respect, honesty, courage, wisdom, truth and humility; and the last seven are for the generations that are yet to be born. Today, in India, it is believed that offering twenty-one stacks of durva pleases Lord Ganesha.

Isn't it interesting that the plants considered sacred always help reduce inflammation? In the same vein, a tree that is considered very sacred is the Arjuna, which is also known as 'guardian of the heart' because of its anti-inflammatory and cardio-protective properties. The story goes that the sons of Kubera, the god of riches, got trapped in this tree for hundreds of years because of their insolence towards Sage Narada. It was only Krishna who was able to release them from this tree and because of this it has been considered sacred.

Arjuna has been mentioned in the Vedas and the three main Ayurvedic treatises, which include the Charak Samhita, Ashtanga Samhita and the Ashtanga Hridayam. In fact, in some texts, it is believed to have originated from the flowers of soma, a plant that is now considered to be extinct. Since then, this tree has been used for various purposes such as in medicine and as timber. Its leaves are used to feed the

SACRED

Antheraea paphia moth, also known as the south India small tussore, which produces the silken strands used to create tussar silk.

The Science

The cooling effect of durva grass is well documented. In Ayurveda, it is believed to be cooling for the whole body. The grass is alkaline in nature and is given to cancer patients by naturopathic doctors. In modern nutrition, it is given to those undergoing chemo. Considering that durva grass has free radical scavenging or antioxidant activity in the range of 60–75 per cent, which is higher than that of Vitamin C, eating this grass has the potential to prevent and perhaps even reverse diseases.

Durva, or doob grass, is one of the best fodder for cattle and it also has an amazing soil-binding capacity. Traditionally, it is used for allergies and extracts of this grass have also shown promise in reducing blood sugar. It contains nutrients such as beta carotene, Vitamin C and selenium, because of which it is deemed effective against allergies in traditional medicine. It is known to calm an upset stomach, soothe inflammation and irritated skin, and cure insect bites and minor wounds. It is commonly planted in lawns, as it grows easily and regrows fast when trimmed. Even if it dries out because of excessive heat, or grazed thoroughly by cattle, this grass can come back to life quickly. That is why this grass also symbolizes fertility, regrowth, purity and prosperity. It is also believed to promote oral health. I don't know about you, but I remember sitting on an open lawn with friends, plucking a blade of grass to chew for its sweet, fresh taste. Even today, I recall its flavour, which for me is reminiscent of a carefree, happy phase, when time stretched out and stress didn't exist in my vocabulary.

In terms of stress, Arjuna is a potent ally to fight against cardiovascular stress. Before there was modern medicine, this tree was also known as the 'god of the heart', as it was used to protect the heart. The part of the tree that is utilized the most is its bark and it has been found that it is antimicrobial, antiviral, anti-inflammatory, antioxidant, anti-allergic and anti-diabetic in nature, with wound-healing and liver-protecting properties. One of its major compounds is 7-methyl-gallate, which is a potent antioxidant found to be beneficial for a wide range of benefits, such as the above. Plus, it also works synergistically with modern medicine to improve its benefits for human beings. But of course, a plant, tree or herb is so much more, with its benefits a combination of various phytochemicals that go beyond a single compound. In addition to 7-methyl-gallate, it contains a high level of flavonoids compared to other plants. This includes triterpenes such as arjunic acid, arjunolic acid, arjungenin and arjunetin; flavonoids such as quercetin and kaempferol; and minerals such as magnesium, calcium, zinc, copper and silica.

There are also small studies that support the benefits of this sacred tree. In one study, 116 participants with stable coronary artery disease who were on medication were given either placebo or 500 milligrams of Arjuna powder twice a day along with their regular medicine. In the participants given Arjuna along with regular medicine, there was a substantial reduction in triglycerides and various inflammatory cytokines after three months. In another miniscule study, eighteen healthy male smokers and another equal number of similarly profiled participants were given either Arjuna powder or placebo in a double-blinded study for two weeks each, after which it was found that there was significant improvement in endothelial dysfunction (a non-obstructive coronary artery disease) after brachial artery reactivity studies. In yet another research, thirty patients with coronary artery disease were given Arjuna powder along with statins for three months which reduced low-density lipoproteins up to 16 per cent, 15 per cent decrease in total cholesterol and 11 per cent decrease in triglycerides. These observances reflect its potential to work along with mainstream drugs to reduce heart disease. However, more research is needed to find out about its long-term side effects, if any.

Application

Durva grass can be easily grown at home and added to your green juices and smoothies and Arjuna chaal can be consumed with both water and milk. A milk-based decoction is preferred in Ayurveda, whereas modern nutrition suggests that the antioxidants in both Arjuna chaal and durva grass are better assimilated by the body with water.

Arjuna Ksheerapaka

Ingredients

100 ml milk
100 ml water
2 tsp of Arjuna chaal powder

Method

Boil everything till it reduces to half. Strain and drink. This is good for those who have heart problems and it also works as a preventative drink for heart problems. You may consume this twice a day or just once a day. This decoction gives strength to cardiac muscles. (Replace the milk with water and boil till it's half the quantity if you wish to consume it with water instead of milk.)

Durva Grass Swaras

Ingredients

1 tbsp grass
1 tbsp water

Method

Mix the grass and water and crush it well together. Strain and drink 1 tbsp in the morning and evening.

....

Drink on an empty stomach in the morning to calm
burning sensation in the body. You can also add other
grasses (wheat and/or barley grass) to this swaras (juice).

....

SHAMI AND BAEL

With leaves that look very similar to the touch-
me-not plant, the shami tree is considered
sacred in India. Worshipping it is believed
to please Shani, the taskmaster planet.
According to an Indian epic, the
Mahabharata, the Pandavas hid their
weapons within a shami tree for a
whole year. The shami tree is also
known as kalpatru of the desert for its
ability to grow in hot, arid conditions.
But that's not all, it produces fruits, a
gum called mesquite and its flowers feed
honeybees owing to its abundant blooms
over long periods of time. When translated, shami means
one that pacifies diseases. It has been prized in Ayurveda for
centuries, with its mentions being made in the Vedas, the
Puranas and in the ancient *materia medica* of India. Even
today, this tree is worshipped, especially on Dussehra, when
its leaves are considered to be like gold or wealth and gifted
with love. It is also considered to be the abode of Shiva. In
fact, one of his names is also Shamiroha, meaning, the one
who goes up the shami tree.

Another tree that is synonymous with Lord Shiva is the bael or bilva tree. It is believed that Shiva resides under this tree; Parvati, his consort, resides in every part of it and the fruits are Goddess Lakshmi's breasts. Lakshmi, who emerged from the mythical churning of the ocean of milk, or Samudra Manthan, is said to have rested on a bilva leaf afterwards. The trifoliate leaves signify Shiva's three eyes and the three functions of the divine—creation, preservation and destruction. Therefore, during the month of saawan (monsoon), when Shiva worship reaches its crescendo, devotees offer the leaves of this tree to their favourite god. The tree is so revered that even a broken branch or fallen tree is not burnt as firewood. This tree was mentioned in the Vedas and the Puranas and can also be seen in the Ajanta cave paintings. Planting and worshipping this tree sanctify the environment around it, not just in a spiritual manner but also because it helps purify the atmosphere by absorbing poisonous gases and neutralizing them.

The Science

The shami tree has rightfully earned its place among the trees that are worshipped. Not only does it boost the growth of the trees growing around it, it also holds the soil and prevents erosion. This tree helps balance nitrogen in the soil and improves its fertility. Farmers use the leaves of this phenomenal tree to fertilize their fields. These leaves also have fungicidal and insecticidal properties that help protect the crops. It flowers abundantly and therefore is a huge attraction for honeybees. The bark of this tree is used to make dyes and fibres, the gum is nutritive, while the flower pods and seeds too are used extensively in traditional medicine. In deserts, the tree's extensive root system stabilizes the shifting of sand dunes. It is used as a windbreaker (barriers used to reduce the force of wind and protect structures) and is often the only plant or tree that provides shade in desert-like, arid conditions, thereby giving travellers the much-needed respite from the heat. It is also crucial to afforestation.

The bael tree of course is highly revered and used in worship but is equally utilized in traditional medicine and folk remedies. For instance, the leaves are used to treat nausea and fever, the bark is used as a remedy for fever and cough, the flower is used to make a tonic for the stomach and intestine, and the fruit is consumed in the hot Indian summer to calm the body and cool it from the inside out.

Nutritionally, the wood apple fruit is packed with vitamins and minerals, such as vitamins A, B and C, plus calcium and phosphorus. Additionally, it has carbohydrates, a fair amount of protein and a large portfolio of antioxidants. This fruit contains the highest amount of riboflavin, also known as Vitamin B_2, which is required for the health of the skin, to form the lining of the digestive tract, for blood cells and brain function. In fact, ripe bael fruit is considered to be a natural laxative, especially when taken in the form of a sherbet. In Ayurveda, the ripe and unripe fruits have different medicinal value. The unripe fruit, when sliced and sundried, is traditionally used as a remedy for digestive ailments due to its astringent taste. The ripe fruit is sweet, aromatic and cooling and is used to increase haemoglobin.

The tree itself is hugely beneficial for the environment. It can easily be cultivated on wastelands or unproductive land. It acts as an absorbent plant that soaks up pollutants and nauseous gases from the atmosphere and makes them neutral. It also comes within the group of plants that work as air purifiers, which give a high percentage of oxygen in the sunlight as compared to other species of plants. Its flowers and volatile vapours deodorize bad odour and therefore this plant is a valuable addition to cityscapes and private gardens.

Application

The easiest way to consume bael fruit is to drink its sherbet. The fruit can also be made into a sweet-and-sour chutney, with jaggery added to it. The leaves can be juiced or added to smoothies. The leaves are good for digestion and have a cooling, astringent effect on the body. If someone has IBS, there is malabsorption; in this case, bael leaves increase the absorption of nutrients. Four to five leaves can be consumed by a person per day. Since the fruit has a hard shell and an extremely soft pulp, it is difficult to eat it as it is. Therefore, it is usually consumed as part of recipes instead of being eaten directly as a fruit. It's not a great idea to consume large quantities of this fruit, as it can cause digestive distress. As for the shami tree, it is wonderful to plant it in front of your house to sanctify and to protect the home and nutritionally enrich the soil.

Bael Sherbet

Ingredients

1 bael fruit
500 ml water
250 ml sugar cane juice
10 ml ginger juice
1 tsp of ground roasted cumin

Method

- Crack open the fruit and scoop out the pulp and soak it in the water overnight. Make sure you mash the fruit into the water and remove any seeds.
- Strain the water to remove the pulp and then boil the water till it reduces to half. Let it cool.
- Then add the sugar cane juice, ginger and roasted cumin. Since bael can cause digestive distress for those with sensitive stomachs, cumin and ginger help make it more digestible. Instead of making a batch of sherbet, it is better to make it fresh every day.

JAMUN AND JACKFRUIT

There was once a beautiful jamun tree right in front of my house. I really loved that tree and used to hug it every morning. It was a large tree, heaving with fruit and was home to many kinds of birds. During summer, children would come to collect its delicious fruit, and it provided shade to municipal workers working in the vicinity. Unfortunately, as is the destiny of most trees in the city, this one too was cut down to build a four-storied residential block. It's been a year since the building was completed, and surprisingly, the tree is still fighting back valiantly because every now and then tiny shoots emerge from the soil—so deep are its roots. But of course, every time the shoots become a bit large, they are snipped down because the residents don't want this large tree destroying the foundation of the building.

Human beings are ruthless not only with fellow humans and nature in general but also plants in particular. There was a time when trees were considered sacred and if any construction had to be done, it was done around the tree instead of uprooting it completely. Today, the only thing sacred are lifeless idols that are more revered than living, breathing trees and animals, which is truly unfortunate. Jamun and jackfruit are some of the most ancient trees of India. In fact, India was once known as Jambuland because of the jamun trees, which are native to the subcontinent.

There are many jamun trees growing around temples, most notably the Jambukeswarar temple in Tiruchirapalli district, in the state of Tamil Nadu. The main deity of this temple is shown sitting under the shade of a jamun tree that protects him during the rainy season. This idol is that of Lord Shiva depicted in his water element. There is much folklore associated with this temple. One legend says that this area became a place of worship after Goddess Parvati came to meditate in the jamun forest near the banks of the river Cauvery and made a Shivalingam from the waters of this river. Another story goes that a sage went to worship Lord Shiva in the mountains and offered him jamun fruits. After Shiva ate the berry, he dropped the seed, which the sage ate, revering it as prasad, or divine offering. The seed sprouted in his belly and soon the tree started growing from inside him. Shiva told him to go to the jamun forest on the banks of the same river that Parvati would come and visit him every day. Eventually the sage grew into this jamun tree and Parvati worshipped the Shivalinga under this very tree, which turned into this temple.

Jamun as a fruit is also called fruit of the gods. It is dear to Lord Krishna, is associated with Lord Rama and its leaves are used to worship Ganesha. It is usually planted near temples because it is considered to be extremely sacred. It is also extensively used in Ayurveda to treat various problems, which range from diabetes to diarrhoea. It is a large, evergreen tree that gives shelter to many birds, animals and insects. Its fruits are eaten by parrots, squirrels and monkeys and it provides a safe space for birds to build their nests. A tree is an entire ecosystem and by cutting down one tree, we destroy the habitats of several species of animals. Of course, this ruthless elimination of trees and with them the natural habitat of animals, birds and insects is affecting us humans and causing climate change.

Jackfruit is another beautiful evergreen tree in which the large fruit emerges out of its stem. It is also commonly seen around temples and gurdwaras and is an abundant source of shelter and food for all species of living beings. Huge trees such as jamun and jackfruit last for centuries. In fact, there is one jackfruit tree in the Mahavishnu temple at Thrikodithanam in south India which is more than 500 years old and has a circumference of about 5 1/2 metres. Legend goes that this tree stands at the exact spot where the idol of this temple emerged out of a fire. There are many other temples that have such sacred jackfruit trees, such as the one in Manipur. Did you know that jackfruit is eaten on Naag Panchami, the day of traditional worship of nagas or snakes, in Bihar? This tree is considered to be so sacred that offering water to it is believed to be equivalent to bathing all the gods. Isn't it interesting how traditional rituals that were about worship actually helped care for and preserve these trees?

The Science

It's fair to assume now that berries of all types are considered superfoods because of their strong antioxidant profile. Jamun is no different. This fleshy berry contains high levels of protein, fibres, vitamins and minerals, such as Vitamin A, Vitamin B_3 and Vitamin C. It also contains anthocyanins (which are found in blueberries), iron, calcium, magnesium, phosphorus, potassium and zinc. This nutritional powerhouse also has a combination of ellagic acid and jamboline, which stops the conversion of starch into sugar, thus making this a great fruit to be consumed to balance high sugar. Jamun seed powder in particular works wonders for this purpose. The fruit is antimicrobial and at the same time works as a prebiotic because of its fibrous texture. Though there are no extensive studies to support the innumerable benefits of this local fruit as compared to, say, a blueberry, there is no doubt that this fruit and the tree are a worthy addition to our diet and community gardens, respectively.

Jackfruit is known traditionally for its ability to control blood sugar. Is the jackfruit a fruit or a vegetable? The beauty of this versatile fruit is that when unripe, it is used as a vegetable in savoury dishes and when it is ripe, it is used as a fruit and in desserts. Because of its fibrous texture, it is also enjoyed in place of meat by vegetarians. Quite often, it is cooked with the same spices used to make meat curries or biryani. It is the largest fruit that grows on a tree and a jackfruit tree can bear anything between ten and 200 fruits, with the weight of each fruit varying from 20 to 50 kg.

This nutritionally dense fruit has been found to be richer than apple, apricot, avocado and banana with regards to certain vitamins and minerals. Plus, it is low in calories. For instance, 100 g contains 94 calories, anything between 287 and 323 milligrams of potassium, and 32–70 milligrams of calcium. It is one of those rare fruits that is rich in B complex, Vitamin C, magnesium, copper and iron. Its Vitamin A content increases as it ripens. Its rich profile also includes a high amount of antioxidants because of which this wonderful fruit has potent anti-inflammatory effects. A lectin known as jackin in the fruit bestows the jackfruit with anti-fungal effects. The leaves, fruits and seeds have also shown antibacterial activity which makes the sacred tree and this humble fruit powerhouse of good health and well-being.

Jackfruit has been termed as the miracle crop by leading food security experts around the world because it has the ability to withstand climate change as compared to other crops such as wheat or corn. The tree does not require pesticides, is drought resistant, has a high yield of fruits through the year and can also grow in degraded soil. These large trees provide shade and shelter, prevent soil erosion and are used to control floods. They are a boon not only to humans but also every species of life. They are truly sacred and worthy of the worship that is bestowed upon them.

Application

It is so easy to make these fruits part of our daily lives. In fact, they already are. We enjoy eating jamun in the summer and jackfruit is eaten all year round. Jamun seeds can also be powdered and eaten. The right dosage is 5 g (1 tsp every day) anytime. But more than the fruits themselves, care must be taken to ensure that the trees too are planted so that not only humans, but also insects, microbes, birds and other living organisms benefit from the roots and canopies of these majestic trees.

Jamun Sherbet

Ingredients

4–5 cups of fresh jamun pulp
Himalayan pink salt (to taste)
Black salt (to taste)
Chaat masala (to taste)
Red chilli (to taste)

Method

Separate the pulp. Do not throw the seeds, instead wash them thoroughly and dry them in the sun. Powder them to use as a nutraceutical since they are very good for balancing blood sugar. Have 1 tsp in the morning with warm water or swirl it into smoothies. Add a bit of jaggery if the pulp is sour, but try to avoid it. Blend in the mixer with the skin on to get a coarse texture and freeze it after adding the above ingredients. Then scrape it so that it gives you a crushed ice texture. If you have molds, you may also use them.

Chakka Puzhukku or Mashed Jackfruit

Ingredients

10 pcs of jackfruit flesh
5 pcs shallots

8–10 curry leaves
½ cup grated coconut
Salt to taste
1 tsp turmeric powder
6 nos green chilli
½ tsp cumin seeds
3–4 tsp coconut oil

Method

- Crush the coconut along with cumin seeds, shallots, green chillies, curry leaves, garlic and two teaspoons of water and keep it separately.
- Remove the seeds and flowers of the jackfruit flesh, clean and cut them into round shape pieces.
- Add the jackfruit flesh into a cooking vessel, add turmeric powder and about 1 cup of water and stir it well.
- Close the cooking vessel and cook on medium flame. When it is cooked well, remove the plate and stir it further.
- Then change some portion of the cooked jackfruit flesh from the middle portion to the side and place the crushed coconut. Cook it further for about 5 minutes on a low flame. After about 5 minutes, add some coconut oil into this mix and stir it well.

PALASH AND KACHNAR

Every year during spring, around the festival of Holi, the palash tree becomes abundant with its flame-coloured flowers. These flowers were used to make colour for Holi by soaking them in water, as this blend is considered to be safe and in fact good for the skin. This tree goes back thousands of years and has also been mentioned in the Vedas as an essential part of yagnas or homa. Some consider it to be a form of Agni Dev, the fire god, while others associate it with Lord Shiva. It is revered by Buddhists as well, as some believe that Queen Mahamaya held on to a branch of this tree as she gave birth to Gautama Buddha. The word 'palash' means 'to have sacred leaves', therefore these divine associations are mandatory.

In the Vedas, this tree has been mentioned as the embodiment of Lord Brahma, the creator of the universe. It has also been mentioned that it emerged out of soma, the divine nectar. Some say it emerged out of the body of Yama, the god of death, whereas others compare its flowers to the red nails of Kamadev, the god of love. It was an essential part of sacrificial fires, or yagnas, and people believed that touching the tree would absolve them of their sins. Though the flowers have no fragrance, they still make for a stunning display of colours. The blooms, which are large and come in bunches, with petals shaped like claws or beaks, make the tree look otherworldly and exotic. In fact, another name for this tree is 'kimsuka', which means 'like a parrot's beak'. With its sacred association and vibrant beauty, it's no surprise that over the years, this tree has been romanticized by poets such as Kalidasa, the fifth-century poet and dramatist.

The Indian subcontinent is full of dramatic flowers, especially when the season changes. Late winter to early summer is marked by the arrival of the divine kachnar, or Indian orchid, a tree laden with these large, vibrant, orchid-shaped blooms that range from a deep fuchsia to pink and white. Unlike the palash flowers that do not have any fragrance, these flowers come with a heady scent that makes them attractive to pollinators and birds. The word 'kachnar' when translated means a beautiful glowing woman, which accurately describes its visually pleasing appearance. In the Vedas, its name was kanchan, which literally means gold. In fact, in some Maharashtrian families, the tradition during the Sahara is to exchange kachnar leaves, which are equated with gold. It's no surprise then that kachnar is also known as sonapatta, which means the tree with leaves of gold. The tree is considered to be special to Lord Vishnu and the white kachnar flowers are offered to Goddess Saraswati, who rules learning.

The Science

Both palash and kachnar trees provide beautiful blooms which in itself should be reason enough to plant these trees.

But that's not to say that they are merely ornamental. The palash, or flame of the forest tree, was used extensively by the tribals in folk medicine. The leaves were used to make cups, plates and wrappers for beedis, whereas fibre obtained from its bark was utilized to make ropes. The tree also hosts the lac insect, which produces the lac gum. Moreover, this tree helps improve the quality of the soil in degraded land as it flourishes on barren land. It helps prevent soil erosion, increases water-holding capacity, has a good carbon-storage capacity and grows in a variety of conditions, such as in swampy, water-logged or commercial lands. It is believed that it can sustain its growth under harsh conditions due to the important antioxidants in its leaves and flowers. This makes palash a wonderful tree for afforestation purposes, as it grows easily, without much care and also enriches the soil quality.

Kachnar is another multipurpose tree and is especially loved by tribals because of its medicinal flowers, leaves and stems and its sacred associations. Its stem, bark and leaves contain an insulin-like protein because of which it is a part of certain diabetes medications. Every part of this tree is bursting with antioxidants and also has antimicrobial properties. It's no surprise then that it was traditionally used for a wide variety of ailments ranging from stomach diseases and insect bites to blood purification. It is also used in skincare. The flowers, which are the most beautiful part of the tree, are edible. Whether you use the buds or petals from the blossomed flower, these are rich in Vitamin C, proteins, fats, carbs and fibre. Of course, this tree is a boon for the environment, as its fragrant flowers attract bees, butterflies and humming bees, making it an important plant for pollinators.

Application

The best way to utilize these trees is to plant them in gardens or within the compound of your home. The trees flower profusely, but they do not become as large as the banyan or peepal tree. The visual display of flowers during changing season will please your eyes and provide food for pollinators. Palash is often used to make sherbet, while kachnar petals are used to make pickles. These recipes help provide us with the potent antioxidants in these plants.

Palash Sherbet

Ingredients

1 cup palash flowers
Ground fennel seeds to taste
Jaggery to taste
Himalayan salt to taste
A large jug of water

Method

Soak all the ingredients in a jug till they lose colour. Then strain and drink. You may add lemon, but that reduces the intensity of the bright-orange colour.

MAHUA AND SAL

In central India, mahua and sal trees are considered to be especially sacred among the tribes. For the tribals, the ultimate deity is nature, which is why these trees are regarded to be worthy of worship. The mahua is worshipped not for its benefits but also because the tribes respect nature for what it is. But as we know by now, every plant and tree has its uses even if they're not discovered or documented yet. Every part of the mahua tree is usable: the flowers, leaves and wood. In earlier times, the tree was also considered to be especially sacred in southern India and was a part of rituals in temples such as the Sri Neelakandeswarar Temple. In fact, the Tamil Saint Valluvar is said to have been born under a mahua tree in the Ekambareshwarara Temple in Mylapore, Chennai. During the Sangam Period, which was about third century BCE to third century CE, mahua oil was used to light lamps in temples. Many kings also planted mahua trees as a gift to these temples, but these days, it is primarily worshipped by the tribes of central India, especially the Santhal tribe, as it is seen as the embodiment of the divine, which watches over them and protects them.

In folklore, this tree is considered to be a kalpavriksha, or wish-fulfilling tree. For the Gond and Halba tribes, mahua helps them build a connection with their ancestors, as they believe that the soul of the dead lives on in nature. For these tribes, religion means nature and before cutting or uprooting any plant, they seek permission, so to say, by offering mahua flowers to the plant. Even before hunting and fishing, these flowers are offered to get permission from nature. The flowers are also used to make indigenous liquor, the flowers and fruits are used as food and medicines, while the seeds and pods are used as fertilizer and also to repel snakes and insects. It is also believed that bears in the forest would get intoxicated by the scent of the mahua tree. There was in fact news of elephants getting attracted by the smell of the indigenous liquor and drinking the liquor after which they slept for hours.

The sal tree is also common in central India and is worshipped by tribes in Jharkhand. It also holds an exalted position among Buddhists. In another version of the Buddha's birth, his mother held on to a branch of a sal tree while giving birth to him in Lumbini, Nepal. Because of this, this tree is often featured in Buddhist shrines and monasteries. Sal trees are part of sacred groves revered by tribals and are a part of their festivals and ceremonies, as the sal tree symbolizes purity and devotion. The Sarhul festival of Bihar is centered on the worship of the sal tree. During this festival, the tree is decorated with flowers, rice and leaves. People gather around the tree to seek blessings for the upcoming year and also offer prayers. The sal tree is also worshipped by childless couples so they can be blessed with an offspring. Indeed, one must learn from the tribes, who love and worship nature and give pause before mindlessly destroying trees and animals.

The Science

It was only until a few decades ago that trees were looked at as keepers of health and well-being, especially among tribals. Trees such as mahua are especially popular because everything from their flowers, fruit and bark to stems is useful for human beings and animals. Mahua flowers, which are naturally sweet in taste, contain a high amount of Vitamin C as well as carotene and minerals such as calcium and phosphorus. They are also excellent for liver health, contain a chock full of antioxidants and are antimicrobial in nature, therefore very valuable. Not only are they utilized as natural sweeteners in food, they are also fermented to make a liquor enjoyed during festivals. Traditionally, these flowers are considered to have a cooling effect. They are also utilized as a tonic to help treat diseases of the skin and eyes as well as blood imbalances and headaches. Because of their cooling and astringent nature, these flowers are especially recommended for people who have high pitta.

The stem of the mahua tree is used as toothbrush sticks to chew on traditionally since it is believed that doing so keeps gums healthy and strong. There is some evidence to support this claim, as these stems were found to have high antibacterial activity and is the best in taste as compared to other traditional toothbrush twigs. Every part of this tree has some sort of medicinal value. The leaf has wound-healing anti-burn properties; the oil is laxative; the fruit is cooling, astringent and works as a tonic; the bark is excellent for itching skin, tonsillitis and stomach ache; and of course, the flower, as we discussed, for its cooling astringent effect on the body. The tree itself has a large, wide-spreading root system that binds onto the soil and helps prevent erosion. It also provides a lot of shade and shelter for birds and animals. What's more is that it can grow on wasteland making it a valuable tree in an age where the soil quality is rapidly deteriorating.

Mahua and sal are usually worshipped together by tribals. The sal tree is known for its durable timber that is resistant to decay. The tree also produces a resin known as guggal, which is used in Ayurveda to relieve bone and joint pain. Locally, it is believed that chewing on a piece of sal tree bark helps prevent dental and gum problems. This tree is considered to be especially hardy against forest fires. It also hosts and supports a variety of flora and fauna, for instance, ground orchids and a variety of lichens. It is home to the Indian giant squirrel and also red weaver ants. Of course, just like the mahua tree, sal too is utilized in traditional medicine, which makes it a huge support for the local population and the environment.

Application

Mahua oil and sal butter are extensively used in skincare. Fresh mahua fruit can be eaten raw or cooked into a halva.

Mahua Ladoos

Here's a simple recipe for mahua flower laddoos, which are good for boosting energy, enhancing immunity and providing essential nutrients.

1. Roast and grind 1 cup mahua flowers.
2. Roast 1 cup coconut and ¼ cup nuts in ¼ cup ghee.
3. Mix with ½ cup jaggery and 1 tsp cardamom. (For the special touch and extra boost, add a spoon of mahua seed.)
4. Shape into laddoos. Ready to enjoy this tribal delicacy.

NEEM AND AMLA

Indeed, the two most useful and popular trees in the Indian subcontinent are neem and amla. They serve a multitude of purposes—from detoxification to building immunity— and it's no surprise that the neem tree is commonly known as the tree of heaven because of its multiple uses. The scientific name of neem is *Azadirachta indica*, which has been derived from the Persian word 'Azad dirakht-i-Hind', which means the noble or free tree because this tree is naturally free of pests. The word 'neem' comes from the Sanskrit word 'nimba', which means the storehouse of good health.

Neem is one of the fastest-growing trees and has been used since time immemorial in our country to heal, cure, protect and defend one's health. Forget about divine associations, the neem tree itself is a goddess by the name of Neemari Devi. In siddha medicine, one of the oldest medicine systems in the world, the first plant ever mentioned was neem, which is also known as margosa. In the Indus Valley civilization, one of the most prominent herbs that was used was neem. Neem has been extensively used in Ayurveda. In fact, almost 75 per cent of all Ayurvedic medicines is believed to have neem as a component. In the Vedas, there is a phrase for neem that says: 'sarva roga nivarini', which basically means one that cures all ailments.

The other tree that rivals neem in terms of its usage and reverence is amla, which is known as the king of *rasayana*, or rejuvenation, in Ayurveda. It is also known as divya or amritphal, which basically means fruit of heaven or the fruit full of nectar. In Sanskrit, it is known as 'amalaki', which translates to 'the fruit where the goddess of prosperity resides'. It is very important in traditional medicine. It is worshipped as mother earth because the fruit is extremely nourishing for mankind.

The tree is considered sacred because it is believed to be the abode of Lord Vishnu. In fact, amla is to Vishnu what rudraksha is to Shiva. On Amalaka Ekadashi, a festival that celebrates the amla tree, the tree is worshipped as a deity itself. In some mythological stories, it is the first tree to be created in the universe.

In another story, it is believed that this tree sprung from the tears of Vishnu, and in yet another version, it is said that this tree originated when the nectar of gods fell on the earth. It is not surprising then that this fruit is utilized by all traditional systems of medicine, including Ayurveda, siddha, unani, Tibetan, Sri Lankan and TCM, to treat a variety of ailments including diabetes and skin disease, and it boosts memory and immunity.

The Science

Both these trees are studied extensively and backed with research that proves their immense medicinal benefits. The neem tree is rich in a variety of compounds that help cool down the body, work against allergies and contain fungicidal and antiseptic properties. Leading the way among these compounds is a triterpene known as nimbin. It is a potent antioxidant that helps reduce inflammation by stalling the production of reactive oxygen species, which basically means an unstable molecule that contains oxygen that easily reacts with other molecules in the cell, thereby causing damage to DNA proteins, lipids, etc. Neem also contains potent flavonoids, which also inhibit reactive oxygen species thereby reducing inflammation. Neem leaf has a particular set of glycoproteins known as the neem leaf glycoprotein, which is a natural immunomodulator that exhibited antitumour activity in mammals. Another constituent is azadirachtin, which is known for its toxic effects on insects. Every part of the neem tree, including the leaves, bark, fruit and gum, has medicinal properties and has traditionally been used to treat conditions such as hypertension, heart disease and diabetes. This is because of their free radical scavenging, detoxifying and DNA-repairing benefits down to the cellular level.

Though neem is a well-known insecticide, interestingly, neem compost was found to be beneficial, as earthworms fed voraciously on it and converted 7 per cent of the feed into vermicompost every day. This compost was made with freshly fallen and partially dried neem leaves interspersed with cow dung and topped up with a layer of fresh garden soil. Environmentally, the neem tree has immense benefits, not least because it is an evergreen tree with a wide root system that grows in dry arid environment, preventing desertification of land. Because of this reason, the neem tree has been planted in several regions in Africa and South America to preserve the land. The tree also has the potential to keep the environment around it cool. A great example of this would be in the Arafat Plains, Saudi Arabia, where 50,000 neem trees were planted in a 10 km sq. area, which provided shade and a cooler environment for haj pilgrims. The neem tree helps absorb carbon from the atmosphere and reduces nitrous oxide in the soil especially when neem seed and oil seed cake are used in agriculture. Incidentally, nitrous oxide has over 2,50,000 times more global warming power than carbon dioxide and it also stays in the atmosphere for much longer.

Another tree that has shown potent antioxidant activity especially to inhibit reactive oxygen species is amla. This is why amla is also another natural food that is great for immunity and is used traditionally for its medicinal properties. It contains a high amount of Vitamin C, which does not degrade under heat or light, because of which amla preparations, such as murabba, pickles and powders, etc. tend to retain the Vitamin C over time. Traditionally, amla has been used to reduce burning sensation in the skin and the eyes, treat anaemia, boost digestion and improve liver health. It also helps tone the cardiovascular system. Amla is a great food to be included in our everyday diet because of its rich profile of antioxidants and phenolic compounds, which are known to have antihyperglycemic, anti-inflammatory and anti-lipid activities. About two or three blueberries are enough to complete the daily requirement of Vitamin C, which just proves that amla has more Vitamin C content than other fruits such as lemon, pomegranate or apples. Its high Vitamin C content is supported by the presence of other vitamins such as A, B_1 and E as well as calcium and iron.

In a clinical study with smokers, it was found that a significant reduction in peroxidation status and increased antioxidants were noticed in people who consumed 250 mg amla twice a day for sixty days. Amla also supports people who have metabolic syndrome. In another clinical trial, people who were consuming either 250 or 500 mg capsule twice a day for twelve weeks showed reduced oxidative stress and increased glutathione levels. In yet another study on humans, it was found that a 500 mg dose of amla extract twice a day for three months reduced total cholesterol and LDL levels in obese people. As for its benefit on diabetic patients, it has been found that daily doses of up to 3 g of amla powder extract reduced blood glucose levels after twenty-one days. But that's not all. The polyphenols from this berry also protect the digestive system by inhibiting a microbe that is a known cause of gastric ulcers. What's more is that the daily consumption of amla extract in the form of a 500 mg tablet twice a day can help reduce the severity and frequency of regurgitation and heartburn in those who have gastroesophageal reflux disease (GERD).

Along with its benefits for consumption, the amla tree is wonderful for the environment especially because it has the potential to grow in degraded areas such as overly mined lands. With such a multitude of benefits for human consumption as well as for the environment, the neem and amla tree have truly earned their sacred status.

Application

Neem was once called the village pharmacy because 110 types of traditional medicines are made out of this wonderful plant. It reduces bugs, eliminates mosquitos and is believed to improve the Vastu of a village. Neem trees were planted as a canopy where village elders sat and smoked their hookahs. The air of this medicinal tree is good for the lungs, and it wasn't planted for godly but for health benefits. The roots of its tree aren't as expansive or destructive as that of banyan or peepal and can be planted around the house. Because it's an indigenous tree, it grows best in temperatures ranging between 14 and 34 degree Celsius. It can withstand the harsh loo wind of the summer and can even survive in temperatures up to 48 degrees Celsius. It grows all over India in various types of soil. Once it is fully grown, it is drought resistant. Interestingly, cows enjoy grazing under a neem tree and chewing on its branch. Neem leaves have been found to have a positive effect on the performance of lactating cows and it can be used for blood purification. Today, Brazil has more desi cows than India. When the cows were transported so were the neem trees. Because of this reason now neem grows in Brazil.

Amla is another tree that can be planted anywhere—from the mountains to the desert and every kind of soil. There are two types of amla: the hybrid variety, which is more common and the wild variety. The former is not strong enough to withstand climate change, whereas the wild variety is from here and is therefore stronger. The root structure of amla is fairly compact, therefore it can be planted around the house.

Neem Detox Balls

Ingredients (for one ball)

1 neem leaf
A pinch of turmeric
1 black pepper
Enough honey to bind

Note: Neem is drying, therefore, if you have a dry constitution, you can't keep eating neem continuously. If you have dryness, consume neem for fifteen days and during that time increase your consumption of ghee.

Method

Crush together and roll into 1 mm or 2 mm balls. Only eat one or two balls at a time. Consume first thing in the morning on an empty stomach. This is good for the immune system, reduces stress and helps purify the blood.

Amla is best consumed as a shot early in the morning. Amla supari, which is basically dried berries, can be eaten any time of the day as a snack. This fruit is the ultimate rejuvenator. Those in the age range of 20–50 years can eat an amla every day. They will look much younger. If you can't get the fresh fruit, then you can consume 5 mg of dried powder anytime during the day.

Amla for Hyperacidity

Ingredients

½ tsp amla
½ tsp licorice powder
1 tiny piece of mishri
1 tbsp ghee

Method

Mix everything together. Chew well and ensure that the saliva has worked through this mixture and only then swallow. This recipe is good for those with hyperacidity.

KADAMBA AND ASHOKA

I am not sure if we've made enough progress or if we are more civilized now than we were before. When man equated nature with the divine in earlier times, it was a more civilized way of living than the way we live now. Trees were considered to be a symbol of fertility and auspiciousness, a mark of divinity, and in some cases, a symbol of love and peace. The kadamba and Ashoka trees symbolize eternal love and freedom from grief. The kadamba is known to be a favourite of Lord Krishna; his romantic tricks with Radha and the gopis often took place in the shade of this magnificent, evergreen tree, with its fragrant blossoms and small fruits that are much loved by animals. This tree is also known as Haripriya, meaning beloved to Hari—another name for Krishna, who is usually depicted as playing his flute under this tree.

In the south, this tree is related to Goddess Parvati, who is said to live within this tree. She provides her blessings in the form of an abundance of fruits. There is in fact an old withered kadamba tree in the complex of the Meenakshi Temple which symbolizes its exalted place in its relation to the goddess. This large tree can be found all across India and plays a critical role in supporting biodiversity by providing habitat for small animals, birds and insects. It's named kadamba after the Kadamba dynasty, as they considered the tree to be holy. Like all sacred trees, this too is mentioned in all Ayurvedic treatises and every part of the kadamba tree from the leaves to its flowers, fruits and even pollen is used to treat a variety of medical conditions.

Another tree that is worthy of note is the Ashoka tree. The name literally translates as 'something that takes away grief'. This too is an ancient tree and has been mentioned in the epics such as the Ramayana and the Puranas as well as Ayurvedic treatises such as the Charaka Samhita. Most notably, the mention of this tree is in the Ramayana, where Sita stays in a grove of Ashoka trees when she is kidnapped by Ravana. It was under the grove of these trees that she first met Hanuman. In yet another story about the Buddha's birth, it is believed that he was born under the shade of this divine tree. In another divine reference, the Ashoka blossom is one of the five flowers on the arrows of Kamadeva, the god of love.

The Science

The truth is that the traditional Ashoka tree, with its bright blooms, is a rare sight these days. However, the False Ashoka tree, which is without blooms, is commonly planted as a bordering tree around gardens and parks and along the roadsides. This tree has immense benefits against environmental pollution. It has a wide, round-shaped canopy and a straight trunk because of which it is preferable in most local compounds. But more than anything else, it works wonderfully to mitigate air pollution. The only downside is that landscapers tend to trim this tree into a very narrow shape. This reduces the spread and density of its canopy which, in turn, diminishes its ability to control air pollution. We should let these False Ashoka trees grow naturally and abundantly as a shield against polluted environment.

The kadamba tree is also beneficial for the environment but in a different manner. This fast-growing, full canopy tree provides shelter for various birds and mammals. When its leaves and fruit drop on the ground and begin to decay, it vastly improves the soil quality of the land under its gigantic canopy. The tree also produces dense clusters of beautifully fragranced flowers, which are a huge attraction for pollinators. Though the tree is considered to be economically important, especially because it is exploited for its wood, and the fruit has immense medicinal properties, yet it is still not valued as a food source. The fruit is rich in zinc, iron, calcium and magnesium and has a high Vitamin C and beta-carotene content. The potent antioxidant and mineral-rich pulp makes the kadamba fruit a functional food.

Application

The truth is that the Ashoka trees we see lining the roads are not the true, native Ashoka. The Sita Ashoka or Desi Ashoka tree, with its vibrant orange blooms that flower in bunches, is almost non-existent today. Therefore, it is a good idea to find this native species and plant it around our homes and gardens. The best time to plant this tree is in the month of August in well-drained, fertile nutrient-rich soil. The ideal temperature is 18–35 degrees Celsius. They need to be protected from frost and should receive up to four to six hours of sunlight every day.

The kadamba tree, on the other hand, is still planted by many. It is excellent for birds because of its small fruit. It is also good to line avenues because of its straight trunk and a canopy, which is not too large even though it's a tall and beautiful-looking tree. The best time to plant this tree is also monsoon. Kadamba grows best in deep, moist, well-drained alluvial soil, which is usually found near the river banks. It requires about six to eight hours of direct sunlight.

TAMARIND

The tamarind tree is the subject of myth and folklore. Some consider it to be the abode of spirits, while for others, it is related to stories of the Ramayana. There are also stories about this tree and its association to Lord Shiva. In Indian mythology, all stories point to the fact that earlier, the tamarind tree used to have big, well-formed leaves. It is believed that Lord Rama took shelter under a tamarind tree when he was banished from his kingdom and was in exile. Since the tree had large leaves, he felt like he wasn't doing his penance correctly. So he asked his brother, Lakshmana, to shoot an arrow at the leaves fragmenting them into the small leaves they are today. In the other story relating to Shiva, it is suggested that the lord himself fragmented these leaves into smaller pieces as a demon was hiding behind its large leaves. Shiva opened his third eye to kill this demon, and the leaves disintegrated into the smaller size as we see today.

A tamarind tree has a lifespan of about 200 years, but there are some that can even go as far back as 400 years. The tree is believed to have originated in India and the word 'tamarind' comes from the Persian phrase 'tamar-i-hind', which basically means the 'date of India'. However, new evidence shows that the tree may have been initially cultivated in Egypt or Madagascar. Before the Spanish brought tomatoes to India, tamarind was used to add a sour taste to Indian dishes. Tamarind is worshipped to this day as a deity by people in rural India and tribal folk and is in fact a huge part of their medical protocol. Tamarind is also used in traditional medicine in western and eastern Africa. As a hardy, multipurpose, drought-resistant tree, it is worthy of worship and a valuable addition to parks and gardens.

The Science

Tamarind is a huge part of India's culinary heritage. It is used to add a tangy flavour to our chutneys and curries. It's a nutritional powerhouse, rich in magnesium, B vitamins, calcium, phosphorus and potassium, as well as all essential amino acids, except tryptophan. The tamarind fruit contains tartaric acid, malic acid, potassium and the soluble fibre pectin, all of which contribute to digestive health and provide mild laxative benefits. The fruit also causes relaxation of smooth muscles, for instance, stomach, intestines, GI sphincters, gall bladder and blood vessels, some on which are also responsible for its laxative effect. But it's not just the fruit but also the leaves of this wonderful tree that have immense benefits. They work as fodder for cattle and in humans the leaves show a liver-protective effect by stabilizing the membranes and decreasing glutathione consumption. The extract from the fruit also decreases fluoride in the plasma and inhibits fluoride-induced liver and kidney damage. Fluoride is found in drinking water and has been linked to several health problems.

The evergreen tree is extremely hardy and grows very well in desert-like areas that are prone to drought. In Africa, it is valuable for wildlife, as it provides shade to animals such as elephants, who can lean against its strong, wind-resistant trunks and branches that can hold the weight of this mighty animal. Locals in Ghana claim that to be safe from an elephant attack one can climb atop a tamarind tree. All in all, the tamarind tree is very beneficial because every part of this tree can be utilized for culinary, nutritional and medicinal benefits. Moreover, it is a hardy tree that has a long life and helps cool the environment in hot, desert-like areas.

Application

Tamarind is best eaten with gur/jaggery, as it takes away the erosive nature of this sour fruit. People who have joint pains may find that their aches and pains get worse when they consume raw tamarind. However, when consumed with gur, it doesn't have this effect, as the sweetness of the gur takes away the pungency of tamarind.

Tamarind Sherbet

Ingredients

1 tsp of deseeded tamarind pulp soaked in water
Jaggery (to taste)
A glass of water
A pinch of pink salt
½ tsp of roasted, crushed cumin

Method

- Crush the tamarind with clean hands into the water that it is soaked in.
- Strain the pulp into the glass of water.
- Add the condiments and jaggery as per taste.
- (This drink is great to enhance digestive fire, cool the body and give a sense of satisfaction, especially during summer.)

CHINAR AND DEODAR

There are mountain ranges all over the world, but the Himalayas are especially sacred. Perhaps it's because of the rishis or sages who walked over these mountains and meditated here, giving the place a special divine energy. There are also associations of these mountains with various gods and goddesses. Or it could be because of the rich biodiversity of the Himalayas, with the variety of medicinal species of plants that gave these seekers food, healing and shelter, thereby energizing their practices. After all, according to the lore of the Ramayana, the mythical Sanjeevani booti was present on Dronagiri Parvat, also known as Mahodaya or Gandhamardan, a mountain believed to be a part of these majestic mountains.

Even today, these mountains are home to various plant and animal species, though not as diverse as a few hundred years ago because these mountains too have been shorn of green cover in the name of progress. Even the most emblematic of trees of the Himalayas—deodar and chinar—are depleting because of the relentless cutting down of these trees. The chinar tree is an emblem of the Kashmir Valley. Chinar—a Persian word that means 'what a fire'—was named so by Emperor Jahangir for its flame-coloured orange/maroon leaves during autumn. It represents Goddess Bhavani and is therefore seen around a lot of temples in Kashmir. Considered to be a gift from heaven to earth, the hollow of the tree was used for meditation by the ancient sages. It is unfortunate that despite its sacred status, about a third of Kashmir's beautiful chinar trees will not survive in the next ten years because of damage due to construction projects. This is why we need to begin the practice of looking at plants and trees as sacred beings and not just from the view point of vegetation. By giving plants divine status, it will perhaps prevent local people from destroying or cutting down these precious trees.

The deodar or cedar is another Himalayan tree that is considered to be worthy of worship, as it was believed that Shiva and his wife Parvati lived among the deodar forests of the upper Himalayas. Because of this reason, the ancient sages used to go into deep meditation within these forests to please the god of destruction. The name 'devdaru' means forest of the gods and deodar is also known as the 'Pearl of Kashmir' due to its abundance in the Himalayan region. Its growth is threatened due to climate change and efforts must be made to preserve this ancient tree, which is a source of cosmetic and medicinal value and of course an integral part of the Himalayan ecosystem.

The Science

Just the fragrance of the majestic deodar tree is enough to transport the mind to a more tranquil space. Now there is some evidence to show that it indeed helps calm anxiety, as seen in animal studies. It has been suspected for a while now that low GABA levels in the brain can be involved in depressive disorders. It was reported in an animal study that deodar extract led to the increase of GABA levels in the brains of rats. Because of this reason, the extract has been found to have somewhat antidepressant, anti-anxiolytic effects in animals through this GABA modulation in the brain. Usually, oil from the heartwood or bark of the tree is used which requires uprooting the entire tree. Thankfully, in these studies, extract from the pine needles was utilized, which are more abundant and a better resource to use, as it leaves the tree intact. It was also found that higher doses of this extract showed a hypnotic effect, which increased the total sleeping time. Research has also found that deodar or Himalayan cedar wood oil has insecticidal properties against mosquitoes, antibacterial effects and anti-fungal effects. Because of this reason, the oil is used topically as an antiseptic, especially in animals such as sheep, goats and camels for the treatment of fungal infections and also as insect repellent.

There is meagre information available about the benefits of the chinar tree. However, because of its large foliage, it can be assumed that these trees provide precious amounts of oxygen to the Valley area. The trees, which are a heritage symbol for Kashmir, have rapidly dwindled in number since the 1970s from about 70,000 to only a few thousand. These dense, green trees need to be protected and vigorously replanted. Though they grow well in riverine soils, they adapt very well to dry soils once they are well established and are capable of living for many centuries growing tall, large and incredibly dense.

Application

No other tree can take the place of chinar and deodar, which are perfect for the temperature and conditions of the sub-Himalayan region. If these plants cease to exist, the mountains will become deserts. After 1990, there has been massive deforestation of the mountains in order to build hotels and restaurants. It is crucial to support and protect these forests, as they are home for the wildlife, such as wolves and bears who, in turn, protect the glaciers and river systems. If these forests are eradicated, wildlife will be eliminated too, which, in turn, will lead to an increase in the goat population that grazes on vegetation. This will lead to further desertification of the landscape that will increase the temperatures of the region, melting glaciers and eventually drying up rivers. We may assume that cutting down trees doesn't affect us, but ultimately this demolition will result in the destruction of mankind. If the constant hurricanes owing to the higher surface temperatures of the sea are anything to go by, we need to stop felling trees and do everything to restore green cover, which is the simplest way to cool down temperatures.

The best time to plant deodar is in spring after the ground thaws during fall before the first frost. The beautiful thing about this wonderful tree is that though it prefers moist, well-drained, slightly acidic, nutrient-rich soil, it can also tolerate a variety of soils, including loam, sand and clay. For this tree, the ideal temperature is 10–21 degrees Celsius and it flourishes in a sunny spot. The best time to plant a chinar tree is during fall so that it has a chance to establish roots before the advent of summer. The best thing you can do to reverse climate change is plant a tree, or at the very least not cut down one, which is infinitely more beneficial for the environment than sipping from a paper straw.

BANYAN AND PEEPAL

There is something about peepal and banyan trees that is incomparable to any other. Maybe it's their aura and energy that calms us when we sit in their shade. Perhaps it is their aesthetic beauty that makes them look ancient and quintessentially Indian.

Or perhaps it's the fact that these trees are the ultimate givers, sharing their massive canopies with a multitude of insects and animals and shade with us humans. And of course, the divine and demonic associations with them make them revered and feared in equal measure. The reason I began writing this book is because of the peepal tree. I wanted to plant it in our community garden but was met with resistance from neighbours and other residents. Some said that even the shadow of this beautiful tree is unlucky for the house, while others said that it would destroy the foundation of their homes. When I researched this tree a little more, I was infatuated with it even more. Perhaps the shadow of the tree is not unlucky, it's a superstition brought about by the fact that it does have a wide root system that indeed can destroy houses and their foundations. Perhaps that's why it is believed that even the shadow of the deep peepal tree should not fall on a house, not because it is the abode of spirits but because of its root system.

It is believed that more than 3000 deities reside within this beautiful tree and that is the folklore I lean towards. I love how the tree sprouts out of the most uninhabitable landscapes, be it a crack in the wall or from the floor made of concrete. When birds eat the small fruit, the seed goes undigested, and when they excrete this fruit, it finds its way into the cracks and crevices of buildings, from where it grows plentifully, even without nourishment. This shows its resilience. Peepal is one of the oldest trees in Indian mythology and scriptures and is mentioned in ancient texts such as the Ramayana, the Mahabharata, the Puranas, the Upanishads, *Arthashastra*, the

Bhagavad Gita and also Buddhist literature. It was known as the bodhi tree, even before Gautama Buddha sat under it, in its shade to meditate and find enlightenment. It is also known as religious fig because it is considered sacred in Hinduism, Jainism and Buddhism.

Despite the reservations people have about growing this tree in their compounds, it is still seen as a symbol of prosperity and good luck and is often planted and worshipped around temples even to this day. One of the longest-living peepal trees happens to be in Sri Lanka which is estimated to be about 1000 years old. Even today, cutting down a peepal tree is seen as a sin, which is why before this tree is cut down or uprooted, a prayer is offered to the tree and only then it is removed from its place of growth. It is the oldest tree depicted in Indian art, with its presence being on some seals from the Harappan civilization. It is also considered to be the tree of the world or the tree of life of the Indian subcontinent.

The peepal tree is supposed to be feminine, and the banyan tree is supposed to be its male counterpart. Banyan is also a variety of fig, just like peepal. Many trees live for centuries, but even the ones that live long, be it peepal or tamarind, eventually die. However, banyan is supposed to be an immortal tree as till today nobody has seen the banyan tree dying unless of course it has been uprooted. For instance, Mylapore in Chennai is famous for its banyan trees; the age of some of these trees is one and a half thousand years. Because of this, it is considered a symbol of longevity and is home to the three main gods: the Trimurti—Brahma the creator, Vishnu the preserver and Shiva the destroyer. The banyan tree has the unique quality of growing in all directions; its ever-growing roots can even grow from the branches of its trees. It is also known as bahupada, meaning 'the one with many feet', because of its innumerable aerial roots. It is also known as the kalpavriksha, or wish-fulfilling tree, since it is believed to fulfill the wishes of the devotees who pray to this tree. In the Gita, Krishna says: 'The banyan tree has its root upwards and branches downwards, the Vedic hymns are its leaves, the one who knows this tree knows the Vedas.'

The Science

The ficus (fig) genus of trees, which includes banyan and peepal, are known to be the most important producer of oxygen, with an excellent photosynthesis rate (the rate of oxygen production in green plant tissues) and also a rich source of minerals in the leaves. Additionally, fig trees are believed to sustain at least 1200 bird and mammal species. In traditional medicine, every part of the peepal tree, whether it's the roots, leaves, stems, fruits or latex, is considered to be therapeutic because of the high concentration of beneficial compounds. The fruits of the peepal tree have laxative properties and are also abundant in antioxidants. Additionally, these fruits are supposed to contain a very high amount of serotonin. The leaves of peepal are considered to have a neuroprotective effect. In small animal studies, it has been found that they help in boosting memory, preventing neurodegeneration and increasing locomotor activity. It's surprising that these sacred trees, which are considered to be so worthy of worship, do not have robust studies and application in modern nutrition.

Environmentally, the peepal tree has a huge number of benefits. In studies done around Pune airport, it was found that this tree was especially resilient to air pollution. In other studies done in Uttar Pradesh, the leaves of this tree were found to be high in heavy metals, especially lead, which also shows its ability to act as a bio accumulator of pollution, meaning that it pulls pollution from the air and in return gives us precious oxygen. This tree is not planted in or around the home because it damages the structure or foundation of a home. However, it is the same wide root structure that can have immense benefit if the tree is planted outside the house, along roadsides or added to gardens and parks because it helps prevent soil erosion. This large, evergreen tree is tolerant to various types of climates, grows in a variety of soil, and has a lifespan of over 3000 years. Thus this precious tree should be cultivated and grown.

The banyan tree is also an excellent ally against pollution. It has a strong root system that helps prevent soil erosion, a wide canopy that makes it home to several species of small animals, birds and bats. Its abundant fruits and aerial branches create a microclimate and an entire world of its own. Like the peepal tree, every part of the banyan tree is considered usable in traditional medicine. However, it is interesting that the aerial roots of a banyan tree are being utilized to create biodegradable fibres that are antimicrobial in nature. The roots of the banyan tree are aerial, which means that creating this fibre does not require uprooting the entire tree. These fibres can be compared to coir and jute, but the real beauty of this fibre is its resistance against bacteria and fungi, unlike other natural fibres because of which they can be utilized in making hygiene products, such as sanitary napkins.

The banyan tree has been employed as a medicinal tree all throughout India and Nepal in various traditions such as Hinduism, Jainism and Buddhism. The banyan fruit itself is a rich source of calcium, iron, potassium and vitamins A, C and K. Parts of this tree have traditionally been used for its anti-inflammatory and pain-relieving qualities. The extract of banyan tree leaves has pain-relieving properties, similar to that of morphine. However, more studies are required for conclusive evidence. Traditionally, a paste of its aerial roots is employed to act against pimples, and the same roots are boiled in oil or water to create a decoction to be used as a hair tonic, and the same roots are also chewed as datuns for better oral health.

Unfortunately, as mentioned earlier, the scientific benefits of these majestic trees have not been studied extensively even though they show immense potential for their medicinal benefits. However, one thing is clear: These trees are certainly an asset because of their environmental benefits. Also, they provide food and shelter to a multitude of animal species and guide us with precious oxygen while clearing the air of pollution.

Application

Peepal thrives best in hot and humid conditions between the temperatures of 13 and 35 degrees Celsius. They require a lot of sunlight and prefer soil that is loose, fertile and well-drained. The banyan tree prefers humid weather but can withstand four to six months of dry weather and do best between 17 and 25 degrees Celsius. They are usually grown in plains and along river banks and prefer well-drained, fertile, nutrient-rich soil. The best time to plant both these sacred trees is between June and September.

These two trees support 150 species of birds and squirrels, small animals, wasps and bees. It is unfortunate that many municipal corporations have banned the planting of these trees because they take up too much space, even though humans have taken over most space across the planet. A single one of these trees is a whole ecosystem in itself. Additionally, a fully grown banyan tree has the potential to support many small businesses. For instance, under the massive canopy of this tree one would find a barber, a small tea shop, a tailor and a few other vendors. Without creating a new structure, using up electricity, or giving rent, three to four businesses would get supported under the shade of this majestic tree. These two trees are micro forests in themselves, meaning that they contain everything that we find in a forest: microbes, insects, birds and mammals.

To support other species is to ensure that we can be safe as humans. If pollinators are not supported, the entire ecosystem will crash because there will be no fertilization, no seeds and no vegetation, leading to the death of herbivores that will lead to the death of carnivores. Think of it this way: if we remove humans, the planet will not suffer. In fact, it is quite the opposite; it will flourish. Therefore, for our benefit (if not for the planet), we must grow, protect, support and nourish plants and trees, which will in turn support other species of insects and animals. So, make space and plant these majestic trees because they will cool down temperatures and support a variety of pollinators and even prevent soil erosion.

Peepal Tree Meditation for Wisdom

- Choose a quiet spot under a peepal tree, ideally one that feels serene and inviting.
- Begin by lighting a white candle near the tree's base—a small gesture to honour the wisdom it holds.
- Sit comfortably and allow yourself a few deep breaths, soaking in the peaceful atmosphere.
- As you meditate, focus on the specific wisdom or guidance you hope to gain, feeling connected to the ancient spirit of the tree.
- Imagine drawing knowledge from its deep roots and expansive branches with each breath.
- When you finish, express your gratitude to the tree for its insights, leaving the candle to burn down fully and safely.

Peepal Leaf Offering for Health

- Collect some healthy peepal leaves, choosing ones that feel vibrant and full of life. On each leaf, gently write a health wish or a loved one's name, using a fine-tipped brush and natural ink.
- Place these leaves in a clay pot filled with water and add a few drops of eucalyptus or camphor oil for their cleansing qualities.
- Position the pot in a sacred space at home, perhaps at your altar. Each morning, as you stir the water gently,

concentrate on your health intentions, picturing healing and vitality encircling the individuals named on the leaves.

- After maintaining this practice for a week, return the leaves to the base of the peepal tree, offering them back with thanks for the tree's enduring strength and protection.

ACKNOWLEDGEMENTS

I couldn't have written this book without the steady and unequivocal support of my publisher and editor. Thank you, Milee and Gurveen, for always supporting my ideas, giving me space and making me feel safe. I feel incredibly blessed to have the support of India's brightest brains. Thank you, Dr Yeola and Lovneet, for supporting me and being a part of my panel of experts year after year. Maneesha for generously donating your family recipes, Dr Cijith for reading and vetting my book and Madhu for sharing your spiritual knowledge. Thank you as well to Peepal Baba, who spent hours with me, talking about trees and their benefits. Also, so much gratitude to Yash Kotak, who provided excellent insights in the cannabis chapter and my friend Dhruv, who always has wonderful suggestions that elevate my book. Thank you to the wonderful chefs Eeshan, Anahita and Pawan for providing me with such brilliant recipes. Sangeeta, Malavika and Rupesh as well for enriching my book with your recipes. Everyone needs support and I appreciate each and every one of you who were there for me. Without you there would be no me or this book.

CREDITS

1. Purification Ritual with Frankincense (by Dr Madhu Kotiya Shezaim)
2. Bhaang Ki Chutney (by Pawan Bisht)
3. Abundance Ritual with Cloves (by Dr Madhu Kotiya Shezaim)
4. Ripe Mango Curry (by Maneesha Panicker)
5. Elá Ada (by Maneesha Panicker)
6. Soothing Coconut and Cucumber Face Mask (by Prakriti Shakti, Kerala)
7. Avial (by Maneesha Panicker)
8. Meditation Bliss Blend (by Sangeeta Jain of Ras Luxury Oils)
9. Awakening Essential Oil Blend (by Sangeeta Jain of Ras Luxury Oils)
10. Pazhamkanji (by Maneesha Panicker)
11. Lotus Root Chips (by Anahita Dhondy)
12. Sesame and Roasted Besan Ladoos (by Malavika Manay of Earth Mama Smoothies, Goa)
13. 'Itminan' Tisane (by Anamika Singh of Anandini Teas)
14. Arjuna Ksheerapaka (by Dr Gunvant Yeola)
15. Bael Sherbet (by Lovneet Batra)

CREDITS

16. Jamun Sherbet (by Eeshan Kashyap)
17. Mashed Jackfruit (by Maneesha Panicker)
18. Palash Sherbet (by Dr Gunvant Yeola)
19. Mahua Ladoos (by Rupesh Pawar, co-founder, Sohrai)
20. Neem Detox Balls (by Lovneet Batra)
21. Amla for Hyperacidity (by Dr Gunvant Yeola)
22. Tamarind Sherbet (by Dr Gunvant Yeola)
23. Peepal Tree Meditation (by Dr Madhu Kotiya Shezaim)
24. Peepal Leaf Offering (by Dr Madhu Kotiya Shezaim)

PANEL OF EXPERTS

Dr Gunvant Yeola, MD, PhD (Kayachikitsa), is an Ayurveda physician as well as principal, professor and head of the Kayachikitsa department at Dr D.Y. Patil College of Ayurveda and Research Centre, Pune. He is also a consultant

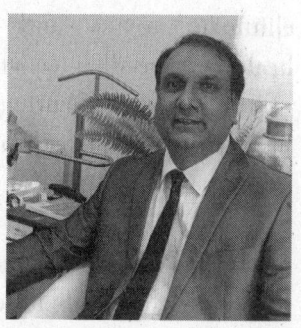

at Vedansh Ayurved and Panchakarma Clinic and Tanman Ayurvedic Research Centre, Pune. He is regularly invited for lectures and consultations in Portugal, the Netherlands, the US and Brazil and is an established name in the world of Ayurveda.

Lovneet Batra is a sports nutritionist who has counselled the Indian boxing, gymnastics, cycling and archery teams during the Commonwealth Games. She is a consultant for the Fortis Group of Hospitals and a visiting faculty at IHM Pusa, New Delhi, in the department of New Product Development and Sports Nutrition. She is the founder of Nutrition by Lovneet and author of *50 Desi Super Drinks*.

Dr Cijith Sreedhar is chief medical officer at Prakriti Shakti in Kerala. As a naturopathic doctor, he believes that the scientific applications of the tenets of natural medicine help eliminate toxins and rejuvenate health. Dr Sreedhar has a track record of healing and preventing diseases in his over seventeen years of practising naturopathic remedies.

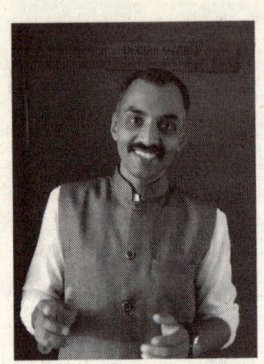

Maneesha Panicker runs Silk Route Escapes, which offers customized, offbeat and luxurious travel solutions across India. She also runs Kayal Island Retreat and Kara Hotel Fort Kochi in Kerala and has an exquisite taste for unusual culinary experiences. In this book, Maneesha has shared several family recipes that blend good taste with health benefits.

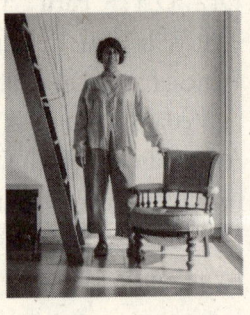

Dr Madhu Kotiya Shezaim is a dedicated practitioner of wicca and is a spiritual healer, psychic and wiccan high priestess, who

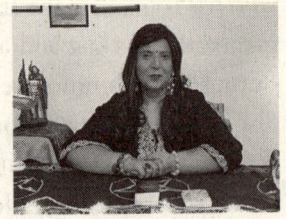

harnesses the power of plants for meditation and manifestation practices. She is the founder of the Wicca India School of Magick & Occult Sciences and director of the MSheziam Institute of Tarot and Divination.

Swami Prem Parivartan, fondly known as 'Peepal Baba', is an environmentalist and the founder of the Give Me Trees Trust, which is the largest voluntary tree-planting movement in India. The trust has over 19,000 volunteers and interns across the country, and together, they have planted over 25 million (surviving and standing) trees in twenty-seven states across the country.

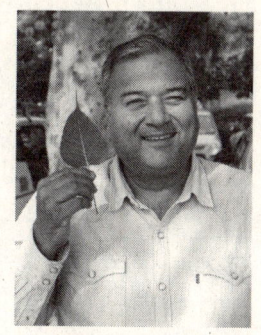

REFERENCES

Introduction

S.K. Jain and S.L. Kapoor, 'Divine Botany: Universal and Useful But under Explored Traditions', *Indian Journal of Traditional Knowledge*, Vol. 6, no. 3 (2007): 534–39, https://nopr.niscpr.res.in/bitstream/123456789/997/1/IJTK%206(3)%20(2007)%20534-539.pdf (accessed on 5 December 2024).

Damian Carrington, 'Deforestation "Roaring Back" Despite 140-Country Vow to End Destruction', *Guardian*, 8 October 2024, https://www.theguardian.com/environment/2024/oct/08/deforestation-destruction-demolition-beef-soy-palm-oil-nickel (accessed on 5 December 2024).

Gayle M. Volk, Patrick F. Byrne and Tara L. Moreau, 'Importance of Plants for Mitigating and Adapting to the Effects of Climate Change', USDA-Agricultural Research Service, Colorado State University, and the University of British Columbia Botanic Garden, https://colostate.pressbooks.pub/climatereadyplantcollections/chapter/importance-of-plants/ (accessed on 5 December 2024).

Martina Egedusevic and Daniel Green, 'Five Surprising Ways That Trees Help Prevent Flooding', Prevention Hub, 18 October 2024, https://www.preventionweb.net/news/five-surprising-ways-trees-help-prevent-flooding (accessed on 5 December 2024).

Afaq Wani, Gyanaranjan Sahoo and Shubham Gupta, 'Sacred Trees of India: Traditional Approach towards Plant Conservation',

International Journal of Current Microbiology and Applied Sciences, Vol. 9, no. 1 (2020): 2606–13, https://www.researchgate.net/publication/344997195_Sacred_Trees_of_India_Traditional_Approach_towards_Plant_Conservation (accessed on 5 December 2024).

PART I

Frankincense and Myrrh

Shimshon Ben-Yehoshua, Carole Borowitz and Lumir Ondrej Hanus, 'Frankincense, Myrrh, and Balm of Gilead: Ancient Spices of Southern Arabia and Judea', *Horticultural Reviews*, Vol. 39, https://naturalingredient.org/wp/wp-content/uploads/1118096789-38.pdf (accessed 12 December 2024).

Aimee Cunningham, 'Incense May Act as a Psychoactive Drug during Religious Ceremony', *Scientific American*, 1 August 2008, https://www.scientificamerican.com/article/mass-appeal/ (accessed 12 December 2024).

H. Hussain, L. Rashan, U. Hassan, M. Abbas, F.L. Hakkim and I.R. Green, 'Frankincense Diterpenes as a Bio-Source for Drug Discovery', *Expert Opinion on Drug Discovery*, Vol. 17, no. 5 (2022): 513–29, https://www.tandfonline.com/doi/full/10.1080/17460441.2022.2044782 (accessed 12 December 2024).

A. Moussaieff, E. Fride, Z. Amar, E. Lev, D. Steinberg, R. Gallily and R. Mechoulam, 'The Jerusalem Balsam: From the Franciscan Monastery in the Old City of Jerusalem to Martindale 33', *Journal of Ethnopharmacology*, Vol. 101, no. 1–3 (2005): 16–26, https://www.sciencedirect.com/science/article/abs/pii/S0378874105002667 (accessed 12 December 2024).

Milica Ljaljević Grbić, Nikola Unković, Ivica Z. Dimkić, et al., 'Frankincense and Myrrh Essential Oils and Burn Incense Fume against Micro-Inhabitants of Sacral Ambients: Wisdom of the Ancients?', *Journal of Ethnopharmacology*, Vol. 219, no. 1 (2018), https://www.researchgate.net/publication/323661383_Frankincense_and_Myrrh_esse

ntial_oils_and_burn_incense_fume_against_micro-inhabitants_of_sacral_ambients_Wisdom_of_the_ancients (accessed 12 December 2024).

Rafie Hamidpour, Soheila Hamidpour, Mohsen Hamidpour and Mina Shahlari, 'Frankincense (乳香 Rǔ Xiāng; Boswellia Species): From the Selection of Traditional Applications to the Novel Phytotherapy for the Prevention and Treatment of Serious Diseases', *Journal of Traditional and Complementary Medicine*, Vol. 3, no. 4 (2013): 221–26, https://www.ncbi.nlm.nih.gov/pmc/articles/PMC3924999/ (accessed 12 December 2024).

Dina E. ElMosbah, Marwa S. Khattab, Shimaa R. Emam and Hala M.F. El Miniawy, 'The Anti-Inflammatory Effect of Myrrh Ethanolic Extract in Comparison with Prednisolone on an Autoimmune Disease Rat Model Induced by Silicate', *Inflammopharmacology*, Vol. 30, no. 6 (2022): 2537–46, https://www.ncbi.nlm.nih.gov/pmc/articles/PMC9700632/, https://egrove.olemiss.edu/cgi/viewcontent.cgi?article=3112&context=hon_thesis (accessed 12 December 2024).

Haritaki

Miaoqing Sha and Baican Yang, 'Haritaki (诃子), Holy Medicine of Buddhism',

Chinese Medicine and Culture, Vol. 2, no. 3 (2019): 141–44, https://journals.lww.com/cmc/fulltext/2019/07000/haritaki,_holy_medicine_of_buddh ism.8.aspx (accessed 12 December 2024).

Kshirod Kumar Ratha and Girish Chandra Joshi, 'Haritaki (Chebulic Myrobalan) and Its Varieties', *Ayu*, Vol. 34, no. 3 (2013): 331–34, https://www.ncbi.nlm.nih.gov/pmc/articles/PMC3902605/ (accessed 12 December 2024).

Shalu Sharma, Bhavna Singh and Hement Kumar, 'A Critical Review of Pharmacological Actions of Haritaki (Terminalia chebula Retz) in Classical Texts', *Journal of Ayurveda and Integrated Medical Sciences*, Vol. 4, no. 4 (2019), https://jaims.in/jaims/article/view/673 (accessed 12 December 2024).

Akhilesh Kumar, Sanjay Kumar, Sapna Chaudhary, et al., 'Encyclopedic Study of Haritaki (Terminalia Chebula Ritz.) In Reference to Prameha', *Journal of Medical Science and Clinical Research*, Vol. 5, no. 7 (2017), https://www.researchgate.net/publication/332012569_Encyclopedic_Study_of_Haritaki_Terminalia_Chebula_Ritz_In_Reference_To_Prameha (accessed 12 December 2024).

Tenzing Dakpa, 'Unique Aspect of Tibetan Medicine', *Acupuncture and Electro- therapeutics Research*, Vol. 39, no. 1 (2014): 27–43, https://pubmed.ncbi.nlm.nih.gov/24909016/, https://glorisunglobalnetwork.org/hualin-international-journal-of-buddhist-studies/e- journal/4-2/1-78/ (accessed 12 December 2024).

Yogesh M. Jirankalgikar, B.K. Ashok and Rambabu R. Dwivedi, 'A Comparative Evaluation of Intestinal Transit Time of Two Dosage Forms of Haritaki [Terminalia chebula Retz.]', *Ayu*, Vol. 33, no. 3 (2012): 447–49, https://www.ncbi.nlm.nih.gov/pmc/articles/PMC3665098/ (accessed 12 December 2024).

E.R.H.S.S. Ediriweera, Peshala Kariyawasam and K.M.S.P. Perera, 'A Clinical Study on Effect of Paste of Haritaki (Terminalia Chebula Retz) in Padadari (Cracked Feet)', *Journal of Ayurveda and Holistic Medicine*, Vol. 2, no. 8 (2014): 2, https://www.researchgate.net/publication/322489532_A_CLINICAL_STUDY_ON_EFFECT_OF_PASTE_OF_HARITAKI_Terminalia_chebula_Retz_IN_PADADARI_ CRACKED_FEET (accessed 12 December 2024).

K.K. Sood and S.Sehgal, 'Cultivation of Superior Harad: A Boon for Farmers of Rainfed Region of Jammu', Early Times, 17 August 2020, https://www.earlytimes.in/newsdet.aspx?q=297405 (accessed 12 December 2024).

Sreelekshmi M., Vimala K.S. and Raiby P. Paul, 'Effect of Haritaki (Terminalia Chebula Retz) with Takra in Dandruff', *Journal of Ayurveda and Integrated Medical Sciences*, Vol. 3, no. 3 (June 2018), https://www.researchgate.net/publication/326430301_Effect_of_Haritaki_Terminalia_Chebula_Retz_with_Takra_in_Dandruff (accessed 12 December 2024).

Sandalwood, Agarwood and Halmaddi

Arlene López-Sampson and Tony Page, 'History of Use and Trade of Agarwood', Vol. 72 (2018): 107–29, https://link.springer.com/article/10.1007/s12231-018-9408-4 (accessed 12 December 2024). Sandeep C. and Manohara T.N., 'Sandalwood in India: Historical and Cultural Significance of Santalum Album L. as a Basis for Its Conservation', ResearchGate, Vol. 10, no. 4: 235–42, https://www.researchgate.net/publication/338434850_Sandalwood_in_India_Historical_and_cultural_significance_of_Santalum_album_L_as_a_basis_for_its_conservation (accessed 12 December 2024).

A.N. Arun Kumar, Geeta Joshi and H.Y. Mohan Ram 'Sandalwood: History, Uses, Present Status and the Future', *Current Science*, Vol. 103, no. 12 (December 2012), https://www.currentscience.ac.in/Volumes/103/12/1408.pdf (accessed 12 December 2024).

'A Synthetic Sandalwood Odorant Induces Wound-Healing Processes in Human Keratinocytes Via the Olfactory Receptor OR2AT4', https://pubmed.ncbi.nlm.nih.gov/24999593/ (accessed 12 December 2024).

'Santalum', ScienceDirect, https://www.sciencedirect.com/topics/pharmacology-toxicology-and-pharmaceutical-science/santalum#:~:text=%CE%B1%2DSantalol%20and%20%CE%B2%2%Dsantalol,oil%20%5B18%2C19%5D (accessed 12 December 2024).

'Clinical Evaluation of Indian Sandalwood Oil and Its Protective Effect on the Skin against the Detrimental Effect of Exposome', Vol. 9, no. 2 (2022): 35, https://www.researchgate.net/publication/359432570_Clinical_Evaluation_of_Indian_Sandalwood_Oil_and_Its_Protective_Effect_on_the_Skin_against_the_Detrimental_Effect_of_Exposome (accessed 12 December 2024).

Manju Sharma, Corey Levenson, John C. Browning, John C. Browning, Emily M. Becker, Ian Clements, Paul Castella and Michael E. Cox, 'East Indian Sandalwood Oil Is a Phosphodiesterase Inhibitor: A New Therapeutic Option

209

in the Treatment of Inflammatory Skin Disease', *Front. Pharmacol.*, Vol. 9 (2018), https://www.frontiersin.org/journals/pharmacology/articles/10.3389/fphar.2018.00200/full (accessed 12 December 2024).

C. Priya and P. Shrikanth, 'Antimicrobial Activity of Ailanthus triphysa (dennst.) Alston against some selected Pathogenic Bacteria', Vol. 11, no. 11(2018), https://rjptonline.org/AbstractView.aspx?PID=2018-11-11-27 (accessed 12 December 2024).

Wang C, Wang Y, Gong B, Wu Y, Chen X, Liu Y, Wei J. 'Effective Components and Molecular Mechanism of Agarwood Essential Oil Inhalation and the Sedative and Hypnotic Effects Based on GC-MS-Qtof and Molecular Docking. Molecules', vol. 27, no. 11 (2022): 3483.

Shui-Tein Chen and Yerra Koteswara Rao, 'An Overview of Agarwood, Phytochemical Constituents, Pharmacological Activities, and Analyses', https://www.traditionalmedicines.org/articles/an-overview-of-agarwood-phytochemical-constituents-pharmacological-activities-and-analyses.pdf (accessed 12 December 2024).

Wen-Yi Kao, Chien-Yun Hsiang, Shih-Ching Ho, Tin-Yun Ho, Kung-Ta Lee,

'Novel serotonin-boosting effect of incense smoke from Kynam agarwood in mice: The involvement of multiple neuroactive pathways', *Journal of Ethnopharmacology*, Vol. 275 (2021), https://www.sciencedirect.com/science/article/abs/pii/S0378874121002968 (accessed 12 December 2024).

Cannabis and Dhatura

G.K. Sharma, 'Cannabis Folklore in the Himalayas', Harvard University Herbaria, Vol. 25, no. 7 (1977): 203–15, https://www.jstor.org/stable/41762786 (accessed 12 December 2024).

Lambert Initiative for Cannabinoid Therapeutics, 'History of Cannabis', *University of Sydney*, https://www.sydney.edu.

au/lambert/medicinal-cannabis/history-   of-cannabis.html
(accessed 12 December 2024).

Marc-Antoine Crocq, 'History of Cannabis and the Endocannabinoid System', *Dialogues in Clinical Neuroscience*, Vol. 22, no. 3 (2020): 223–28, https://pmc.ncbi.nlm.nih.gov/articles/PMC7605027/ (accessed 12 December 2024).

Mark S. Ferrara, 'Peak-Experience and the Entheogenic Use of Cannabis in World Religions', *Journal of Psychedelic Studies,* Vol. 4, no. 3 (2020), https://www.researchgate.net/publication/347574314_Peak-experience_and_the_entheogenic_use_of_cannabis_in_world_religions (accessed 12 December 2024).

Bulcsu Siklós, 'Datura Rituals in the Vajramahabhairava-Tantra', *Acta Orientalia Academiae Scientiarum Hungaricae*, Vol. 47, no. 3 (1994): 409–16, https://www.jstor.org/stable/23658487 (accessed 12 December 2024).

R. Geeta and Waleed Gharaibeh, 'Historical evidence of Datura in the Old World and implications for a first millennium transfer from the New World', *Journal of Biosciences*, Vol. 32, no. 7: 1227–44, https://www.researchgate.net/publication/5649991_Historical_evidence_of_Datura_in_the_Old_World_and_implications_for_a_first_millennium_transfer_from_the_New_World#pf11 (accessed 12 December 2024).

Richard B. Applegate, 'The Datura Cult Among the Chumash', *Journal of California Anthropology*, Vol. 2, no. 1, https://escholarship.org/content/qt37r1g44r/qt37r1g44r.pdf (accessed 12 December 2024).

Dante F. Placido and Charles C. Lee, 'Potential of Industrial Hemp for Phytoremediation of Heavy Metals', *Plants (Basel)*, Vol. 11, no. 5 (2023, :595, https://pmc.ncbi.nlm.nih.gov/articles/PMC8912475/ (accessed 12 December 2024).

Prakat Karki and Madhavi Rangaswamy, 'A Review of Historical Context and Current Research on Cannabis Use in India', *Indian Journal of Psychological Medicine,* https://pmc.ncbi.nlm.nih.gov/articles/PMC10011848/ (accessed 12 December 2024).

REFERENCES

Kevin Hill and Michael Hsu, 'Cognitive Effects in Midlife of Long-Term Cannabis Use', 14 June 2022, Harvard Health Publishing, https://www.health.harvard.edu/blog/cognitive-effects-of-long-term-cannabis-use-in-midlife-202206142760 (accessed 12 December 2024).

Dr Swapna Swayamprava, Dr Subrat Kumar Ojha and Dr Niranjan S., 'Role of Dhatura Patra Swarasa in the Management of Indralupta (Alopecia Areata)', *World Journal of Pharmaceutical and Life Sciences*, Vol. 6, no. 9 (2020): 173–77, https://www.wjpls.org/download/article/56082020/1598852728.pdf (accessed 12 December 2024).

W.F. Mueller, G.W. Bedell, S. Shojaee and P.J. Jackson, 'Bioremediation of TNT Wastes by Higher Plants', National Laboratories, Life Sciences Division, https://engg.k-state.edu/hsrc/95Proceed/mueller.pdf (accessed 12 December 2024).

Cinnamon, Cloves and Bay Leaf

Pallavi Kawatra and Rathai Rajagopalan, 'Cinnamon: Mystic Powers of a Minute Ingredient', *Pharmacognosy Research*, Vol. 7 (Suppl 1, 2015): S1–S6, https://www.ncbi.nlm.nih.gov/pmc/articles/PMC4466762/ (accessed 12 December 2024).

Rohitha Dasanayaka, 'Cinnamon: A Spice of an Indigenous Origin—Historical Study', ResearchGate, March 2019, https://www.researchgate.net/publication/331588549_Cinnamon_A_Spice_of_an_Ind igenous_Origin-_Historical_Study (accessed 12 December 2024).

Saima Batool et al., 'Bay Leaf', *Medicinal Plants of South Asia*, ed. Muhammad Asif Hanif et al., September 2019: 63–74, https://pmc.ncbi.nlm.nih.gov/articles/PMC7152419/ (accessed 29 January 2025).

Haralampos Harissis, 'A Bittersweet Story: The True Nature of the Laurel of the Oracle of Delphi', *Perspectives in Biology and Medicine*, Vol. 57, no. 3 (June 2014): 351–60, https://www.researchgate.net/publication/276147773_A_Bittersweet_Story_The_True_Nature_of_the_Laurel_of_the_Oracle_of_Delphi (accessed 29 January 2025).

Milda E. Embuscado, 'Spices and Herbs: Natural Sources of Antioxidants: A Mini Review', *Journal of Functional Foods*, Vol. 18, Part B (October 2015): 811–19, https://www.sciencedirect.com/science/article/pii/S1756464615001127 (accessed 29 January 2025).

Ankit Shukla and Nagendra Yadav, 'Role of Indian Spices in Indian History', *International Journal of Management Research and Review*, Vol. 8, no. 11 (2018): 1–6, https://www.researchgate.net/publication/365451144_ROLE_OF_INDIAN_SPICES_IN_INDIAN_HISTORY (accessed 12 December 2024).

Lalith Suriyagoda et al., '"Ceylon Cinnamon": Much More Than Just a Spice', *Plants, People, Planet*, Vol. 3, no. 4 (April 2021): 319–36, https://nph.onlinelibrary.wiley.com/doi/full/10.1002/ppp3.10192 (accessed 29 January 2025).

Charu Gupta et al., 'Comparative Study of Cinnamon Oil and Clove Oil on Some Oral Microbiota', *Acta Bio-Medica: Atenei Parmensis*, Vol. 82, no. 3 (December 2011): 197–99, https://www.researchgate.net/publication/229073095_Comparative_study_of_cinnam on_oil_and_clove_oil_on_some_oral_microbiota (accessed 12 December 2024).

Sedigheh Bakhtiari et al., 'The Effects of Cinnamaldehyde (Cinnamon Derivatives) and Nystatin on *Candida Albicans* and *Candida Glabrata*', *Open Access Macedonian Journal of Medical Sciences*, Vol. 7, no. 7 (April 2019): 1067–70, https://www.ncbi.nlm.nih.gov/pmc/articles/PMC6490497/#:~:text=Cinnamaldehyde%20extract%20at%20a%20concentration,the%20loss%20of%20Candida%20glabrata (accessed 29 January 2025).

Alejandra Ponce, Sara I. Roura and María del R. Moreira, 'Essential Oils as Biopreservatives: Different Methods for the Technological Application in Lettuce Leaves', *Journal of Food Science*, Vol. 76, no. 1 (2011): M34–40, https://pubmed.ncbi.nlm.nih.gov/21535691/ (accessed 29 January 2025).

María G. Goñi et al., 'Chapter 39: Clove (*Syzygium aromaticum*) Oils', *Essential Oils in Food Preservation, Flavor and Safety*, 2016: 349–57, https://www.sciencedirect.com/science/article/abs/pii/B9780124166417000390 (accessed 29 January 2025).

Amit Krishna De and Minakshi De, 'Chapter 28: Functional and Therapeutic Applications of Some General and Rare Spices', *Functional Foods and Nutraceuticals in Metabolic and Non-Communicable Diseases*, 2022: 411–20, https://www.sciencedirect.com/science/article/abs/pii/B9780128198155000446 (accessed 29 January 2025).

Vinay Kumar Pandey et al., 'A Comprehensive Review on Clove (*Caryophyllus aromaticus L.*) Essential Oil and Its Significance in the Formulation of Edible Coatings for Potential Food Applications', *Frontiers in Nutrition*, Vol. 9, September 2022, https://www.frontiersin.org/journals/nutrition/articles/10.3389/fnut.2022.987674/full (accessed 29 January 2025).

Milind Parle and Deepa Khanna, 'Clove: A Champion Spice', *International Journal of Research in Ayurveda and Pharmacy*, Vol. 2, no. 1 (November 2010), https://www.researchgate.net/publication/267402397_Clove_A_champion_spice (accessed 29 January 2025).

Shelley Wood, 'Cinnamon and Cloves: Benefits in Diabetes Probed', Medscape, 4 April 2006, https://www.medscape.com/viewarticle/788348?form=fpf (accessed 29 January 2025).

Keith Singletary, 'Bay Leaf: Potential Health Benefits', *Nutrition Today*, Vol. 56, no. 4 (July/August 2021): 202–08, https://journals.lww.com/nutritiontodayonline/Fulltext/2021/07000/Bay_Leaf__Potential_Health_Benefits.8.aspx# (accessed 29 January 2025).

Ion Brinza et al., 'Bay Leaf (*Laurus Nobilis L.*) Incense Improved Scopolamine-Induced Amnesic Rats by Restoring Cholinergic Dysfunction and Brain Antioxidant Status', *Antioxidants*, Vol. 10, no. 2 (2021): 259, https://www.mdpi.com/2076-3921/10/2/259 (accessed 29 January 2025).

Maedeh Ghovvati et al., 'Efficacy of Topical Cinnamon Gel for the Treatment of Facial Acne Vulgaris: A Preliminary Study', *Biomedical Research and Therapy*, Vol. 6, no. 1 (2019): 2958–65, http://bmrat.org/index.php/BMRAT/article/view/515 (accessed 29 January 2025).

K.S. Misar et al., 'Formulation and Evaluation of Antiacne Cream by Using Clove Oil', *Materials Today Proceedings*,

Vol. 29, no. 9 (July 2020), https://www.researchgate.net/publication/342809650_Formulation_and_evaluation_of_antiacne_cream_by_using_Clove_oil (accessed 29 January 2025).

Saffron and Camphor

Mohammad Hossein et al., 'The Ocular Hypotensive Effect of Saffron Extract in Primary Open Angle Glaucoma: A Pilot Study', *BMC Complementary and Alternative Medicine*, Vol. 14, October 2014, https://pmc.ncbi.nlm.nih.gov/articles/PMC4213480/ (accessed 29 January 2025).

Mohammad J Siddiqui et al., 'Saffron (*Crocus sativus* L.): As an Antidepressant', *Journal of Pharmacy and Bioallied Sciences*, Vol. 10, no. 4 (2018): 173–80, https://pmc.ncbi.nlm.nih.gov/articles/PMC6266642/ (accessed 29 January 2025).

Alireza Lashay et al., 'Short-Term Outcomes of Saffron Supplementation in Patients with Age-Related Macular Degeneration: A Double-Blind, Placebo-Controlled, Randomized Trial', *Medical Hypothesis, Discovery & Innovation Ophthalmology Journal*, Vol. 5, no. 1 (2016): 32–38, https://pmc.ncbi.nlm.nih.gov/articles/PMC5342880/ (accessed 29 January 2025).

Jia Xiong et al., 'Evaluation of Saffron Extract Bioactivities Relevant to Skin Resilience', *Journal of Herbal Medicine*, Vol. 37, February 2023, https://www.sciencedirect.com/science/article/abs/pii/S2210803323000076?via%3Dihub (accessed 29 January 2025).

Paolo Zuccarini, 'Camphor: Benefits and Risks of a Widely Used Natural Product', *Acta Biologica Szegediensis*, Vol. 53, no. 2 (January 2009): 77–82, https://www.researchgate.net/publication/236017993_Camphor_Benefits_and_risks_of_a_widely_used_natural_product (accessed 29 January 2025).

J.T. Fu et al., 'Fumigant Toxicity and Repellence Activity of Camphor Essential Oil from *Cinnamonum camphora* Siebold Against *Solenopsis invicta* Workers (Hymenoptera:Formicidae)', *Journal of Insect Science*, Vol. 15, no. 1 (September 2015), https://pmc.ncbi.nlm.nih.gov/articles/PMC4664941/ (accessed 29 January 2025).

Mohamed Joonus Aynul Fazmiya et al., 'Current Insights on Bioactive Molecules, Antioxidant, Anti-Inflammatory, and Other Pharmacological Activities of Cinnamomum camphora Linn', *Oxidative Medicine and Cellular Longevity*, ed. Tarique Hussain, Vol. 2022, no. 1 (October 2022), https://onlinelibrary.wiley.com/doi/10.1155/2022/9354555 (accessed 29 January 2025).

Aabid M. Rather, 'Saffron Cultivation in Kashmir Valley: Myth and Realities', *Science and Culture*, Vol. 80, no. 3–4 (January 2014): 68–70, https://www.researchgate.net/publication/317006500_Saffron_Cultivation_in_Kashmir_Valley-Myth_and_Realities (accessed 12 December 2024).

Tibor Wenger, 'History of Saffron', *Longhua Chinese Medicine*, Vol. 5, June 2022, https://cdn.amegroups.cn/journals/ales/files/journals/32/articles/8189/public/8189-PB4-2616-R4.pdf (accessed 29 January 2025).

James McHugh, 'From Precious to Polluting: Tracing the History of Camphor in Hinduism', *Material Religion*, Vol. 10, no. 1 (2014): 30–53, https://www.tandfonline.com/doi/abs/10.2752/175183414X13909887177501 (accessed 29 January 2025).

Renu Dixit, Gudi Lalitha and K.V.V. Bhaskara Reddy, 'A Comprehensive Ayurvedic Literary Review of Karpura', *International Journal of Pharmaceutical Research and Applications*, Vol. 7, no. 3 (2022): 1066–81, https://ijprajournal.com/issue_dcp/A%20Comprehensive%20Ayurvedic%20Literary%20Review%20Of%20Karpura.pdf (accessed 12 December 2024).

Brahmi and Gotu Kola

James M. Brimson et al., 'The Effectiveness of *Bacopa monnieri* (Linn.) *Wettst.* as a Nootropic, Neuroprotective, or Antidepressant Supplement: Analysis of the Available Clinical Data', *Scientific Reports*, Vol. 11, January 2021, https://

www.nature.com/articles/s41598-020-80045-2 (accessed 12 December 2024).

Raimondo Gaglio et al., 'Effect of Saffron Addition on the Microbiological, Physicochemical, Antioxidant and Sensory Characteristics of Yoghurt', *International Journal of Dairy Technology*, Vol. 72, no. 2 (November 2018): 208–17, https://www.researchgate.net/publication/328932825_Effect_of_saffron_addition_on_the_microbiological_physicochemical_antioxidant_and_sensory_characteristics_of_ yoghurt (accessed 12 December 2024).

Navneet Kumar et al., 'Efficacy of Standardized Extract of *Bacopa monnieri* (Bacognize®) on Cognitive Functions of Medical Students: A Six-Week, Randomized Placebo-Controlled Trial', *Evidence-Based Complementary and Alternative Medicine*, Vol. 2016, no. 1 (October 2016), https://pmc.ncbi.nlm.nih.gov/articles/PMC5075615/ (accessed 29 January 2025).

Steven Roodenrys et al., 'Chronic Effects of Brahmi (*Bacopa monnieri*) on Human Memory', *Neuropsychopharmacology*, Vol. 27, no. 2 (August 2002): 279–81, https://pubmed.ncbi.nlm.nih.gov/12093601/ (accessed 12 December 2024).

James D. Kean et al., 'A Randomized Controlled Trial Investigating the Effects of a Special Extract of *Bacopa monnieri* (CDRI 08) on Hyperactivity and Inattention in Male Children and Adolescents: BACHI Study Protocol (ANZCTRN12612000827831)', *Nutrients*, Vol. 7, no. 12 (2015): 9931–45, https://www.mdpi.com/2072-6643/7/12/5507 (accessed 29 January 2025).

Jatuporn Phoemsapthawee et al., 'Does Gotu Kola Supplementation Improve Cognitive Function, Inflammation, and Oxidative Stress More Than Multicomponent Exercise Alone? – A Randomized Controlled Study', *Journal of Exercise Rehabilitation*, Vol. 18, no. 5 (October 2022): 330–42, https://pmc.ncbi.nlm.nih.gov/articles/PMC9650315/ (accessed 29 January 2025).

Sebastian Aguiar and Thomas Borowski, 'Neuropharmacological Review of the Nootropic Herb *Bacopa monnieri*', *Rejuvenation Research*, Vol. 16, no. 4 (August 2013): 313–26, https://pmc.

ncbi.nlm.nih.gov/articles/PMC3746283/#:~:text=The%20
herb%20was%20allegedly%20used,Centella%20asiatica%20
(Gotu%20Kola) (accessed 29 January 2025).

PART II

Paan and Miswak

Niranjan Chandra Shah, 'Betel Industry in India & South and South
East Asia: The History of Areca catechu (Betel-nut, supari)
& Piper betel (Betel-leaf, Pan) in India (Part I-V)', *Scitech
Journal*, Vol. 2, no. 5-9 (2015), https://www.researchgate.net/
publication/377979239_Feature_Article_Betel_Industry_in_
India_South_and_South_East_Asia_The_History_of_Areca_
catechuBetel-nut_supari_Piper_betel_Betel-leaf_Pan_in_
India_Part_I_-V (accessed 30 January 2025).

Sushil Kumar and Vidyanath Jha, 'Betel (*Piper betle*) as a Basis of
Oral and Digestive Health Security – A Case Study of Mithila
Region in North Bihar, India', *Flora and Fauna*, Vol. 30, no.
1 (2024): 23–28, http://floraandfona.org.in/Uploaded%20
Pdf/301/23-28.pdf (accessed 30 January 2025).

Rakesh Kumar Gupta, Proshanta Guha and Prem Prakash Srivastav,
'Phytochemical and Biological Studies of Betel Leaf (*Piper betle*
L.): Review on Paradigm and Its Potential Benefits in Human
Health', *Acta Ecologica Sinica*, Vol. 43, no. 5 (October 2023):
721–32, https://www.sciencedirect.com/science/article/abs/
pii/S1872203222000713 (accessed 30 January 2025).

Devyani Chandrakant Kirve, 'An Overview of Betel Leaf: Green
Gold of India', *Journal of Pharmacognosy and Phytochemistry*,
Vol. 13, no. 2 (2024): 240–48, https://www.phytojournal.
com/archives/2024/vol13issue2/PartC/13-2-21-577.pdf
(accessed 12 December 2024).

Suboh Aziz Natnoo, 'Betel-Leaf (Pan) Culture: A Study of
Mughal India', *SSRG International Journal of Humanities
and Social Science*, Vol. 5, no. 1 (2018): 39–41, https://www.
internationaljournalssrg.org/IJHSS/2018/Volume5-Issue1/
IJHSS-V5I1P107.pdf (accessed 12 December 2024).

Subhash Chander Ahuja and Uma Ahuja, 'Betel Leaf and Betel Nut in India: History and Uses', *Asian Agri-History*, Vol. 15, no. 1 (2011): 13–35, https://www.researchgate.net/publication/292469329_Betel_leaf_and_betel_nut_in_India_History_and_uses#:~:text=The%20exchange%20of%20betel%20leaves,sign%20of%20marriage%20or%20betrothal. (accessed 30 January 2025).

Akhter Husain and Salman Khan, 'Miswak: The Miracle Twig', *Archives of Medicine and Health Sciences*, Vol. 3, no. 1 (2015): 152–54, https://journals.lww.com/armh/fulltext/2015/03010/miswak__the_miracle_twig.34.aspx (accessed 30 January 2025).

Shaykh-e-Tareeqat and Ameer-e-Ahl-e-Sunnat, *Virtues of Miswak* (2016), translated by Majlis-e-Tarajim (Dawat-e-Islami), https://www.scribd.com/document/369734822/Virtues-of-Miswak (accessed 30 January 2025).

Basil H. Aboul-Enein, 'The Miswak (*Salvadora persica L.*) Chewing Stick: Cultural Implications in Oral Health Promotion', *Saudi Journal for Dental Research*, Vol. 5, no.1 (2014): 9–13, https://www.sciencedirect.com/science/article/pii/S2210815713000188 (accessed 30 January 2025).

Mango and Banana

Marianna Lauricella et al., 'Multifaceted Health Benefits of *Mangifera indica* L. (Mango): The Inestimable Value of Orchards Recently Planted in Sicilian Rural Areas', *Nutrients*, Vol. 9, no. 5, May 2017, https://pmc.ncbi.nlm.nih.gov/articles/PMC5452255/ (accessed 30 January 2025).

Maria Elena Maldonado-Celis et al., 'Chemical Composition of Mango (*Mangifera indica* L.) Fruit: Nutritional and Phytochemical Compounds', *Frontiers in Plant Science*, Vol. 10, October 2019, https://pmc.ncbi.nlm.nih.gov/articles/PMC6807195/ (accessed 30 January 2025).

Pia Asuncion et al., 'The Effects of Fresh Mango Consumption on Gut Health and Microbiome – Randomized Controlled Trial', *Food Science & Nutrition*, Vol. 11, no. 4 (February

REFERENCES

2023): 2069–78, https://pmc.ncbi.nlm.nih.gov/articles/PMC10084975/ (accessed 30 January 2025).

Yanni Papanikolaou and Victor L. Fulgoni III, 'Mango Consumption is Associated with Improved Nutrient Intakes, Diet Quality, and Weight-Related Health Outcomes', *Nutrients*, ed. Gary Wil-liamson, Vol. 14, no. 1 (December 2021), https://pmc.ncbi.nlm.nih.gov/articles/PMC8746860/ (accessed 30 January 2025).

Fatima Zahra et al., 'Health Benefits of Banana (*Musa*): A Review Study," *International Journal of Biosciences*, Vol. 18, no. 4 (2021): 189–99, https://www.researchgate.net/publication/352793672_Health_benefits_of_banana_Musa-_A_review_study (accessed 12 December 2024).

Payal Kumari, Supriya S. Gaur and Ravindra K. Tiwari, 'Banana and Its By-Products: A Comprehensive Review on Its Nutritional Composition and Pharmacological Benefits', *eFood*, Vol. 4, no. 5 (September 2023): 1–23, https://www.researchgate.net/publication/373921417_Banana_and_its_by-products_A_comprehensive_review_on_its_nutritional_composition_and_pharmacological_benefits (accessed 30 January 2025).

Nitamani Choudhury, C. Nickhil and Sankar Chandra Deka, 'Comprehensive Review on the Nutritional and Therapeutic Value of Banana By-Products and Their Applications in Food and Non-Food Sectors', *Food Bioscience*, Vol. 56, December 2023, https://www.sciencedirect.com/science/article/abs/pii/S2212429223010672?via%3Dihub (accessed 30 January 2025).

Deependra Yadav and S.P. Singh, 'Mango: History, Origin and Distribution', *Journal of Pharmacognosy and Phytochemistry*, Vol. 6, no. 6 (2017): 1257–62, https://www.phytojournal.com/archives/2017/vol6issue6/PartR/6-6-82-484.pdf (accessed 12 December 2024).

Jujube and Coconut

Department of Social Forestry Commission, J&K, 'Sacred Groves and Heritage Trees of Jammu and Kashmir', https://jksocialforestry.

in/forestry/forestry/orders/Sacred%20Groves%20and%20 Heritage%20Trees%20of%20Jammu%20and%20Kashmir. pdf (accessed 12 December 2024).

Mengjun Liu et al., 'The Historical and Current Research Progress on Jujube – A Superfruit for the Future', *Horticulture Research*, Vol. 7, August 2020, https://www.nature.com/articles/ s41438-020-00346-5 (accessed 12 December 2024).

Amots Dafni, Shay Levy and Efraim Lev, 'The Ethnobotany of Christ's Thorn Jujube (*Ziziphus spina-christi*) in Israel', *Journal of Ethnobiology and Ethnomedicine*, Vol. 1, September 2005, https://ethnobiomed.biomedcentral.com/ articles/10.1186/1746-4269-1-8 (accessed 30 January 2025).

Subhash Chander Ahuja, Siddharth Ahuja and Uma Ahuja, 'Coconut: History, Uses, and Folklore', *Asian Agri-History*, Vol. 18, no. 3 (2014): 221–48, https://www.researchgate. net/publication/290976239_Coconut_-_History_uses_and_ folklore (accessed 12 December 2024).

Lisa Matricciani et al., 'Branched-Chain Amino Acids and Sleep: A Population-Derived Study of Australian Children Aged 11–12 Years and Their Parents', *Journal of Sleep Research*, Vol. 32, no. 4 (February 2023), https://onlinelibrary.wiley.com/ doi/full/10.1111/jsr.13855#:~:text=Micronutrients%2C%20 particularly%20amino%20acids%2C%20are,across%20 the%20blood%E2%80%93brain%20barrier (accessed 30 January 2025).

Yang Lu et al., 'Research Advances in Bioactive Components and Health Benefits of Jujube (*Ziziphus jujuba* Mill.) Fruit', *Journal of Zhejiang University – Science B*, Vol. 22, June 2021: 431– 49, https://pmc.ncbi.nlm.nih.gov/articles/PMC8214949/ (accessed 30 January 2025).

T. Rajamohan and U. Archana, 'Nutrition and Health Aspects of Coconut', *The Coconut Palm (Cocos nucifera L.) – Research and Development Perspectives*, January 2018: 757–77, https://www. researchgate.net/publication/331136850_Nutrition_and_ Health_Aspects_of_Coconut (accessed 12 December 2024).

Upali Samarajeewa, 'Coconut: Nutritional and Industrial Significance', *Nut Consumption and Its Usefulness in the*

Modern World, ed. Romina Alina Vlaic Marc et al., 2024, https://www.intechopen.com/chapters/1179190 (accessed 30 January 2025).

J.S. Bal, D.R. Sharma and P. Singh, 'Historic *Ber* (Jujube) Trees in Golden Temple, Amritsar (Punjab) – Twenty Years of Consistent Care', *II International Jujube Symposium*, Vol. 1, May 2013, https://www.actahort.org/books/993/993_4.htm (accessed 30 January 2025).

Ranil Jayawardena et al., 'Health Effects of Coconut Oil: Summary of Evidence from Systematic Reviews and Meta-Analysis of Interventional Studies', *Diabetes & Metabolic Syndrome: Clinical Research & Reviews*, Vol. 15, no. 2 (2021): 549–55, https://www.sciencedirect.com/science/article/abs/pii/S187140212100062X (accessed 30 January 2025).

Jasmine and Parijat

T. Gobinath, 'Madurai Malli: The Fragrant Essence of Madurai', *Journal of Emerging Technologies and Innovative Research*, Vol. 11, no. 1 (2024): 170–76, https://www.jetir.org/papers/JETIR2401716.pdf (accessed 12 December 2024).

Uma Kannan, *Madurai Malligai: Madurai and Its Jasmine – A Celebration*, ed. Veena Seshadri (Madurai: Thiagarajar College, Publication Division, 2012).

Vidyavati Hiremath et al., 'Literary Review of Parijata (*Nyctanthus Arbor-Tristis* Linn.) An Herbal Medicament with Special Reference to Ayurveda and Botanical Literatures', *Biomedical and Pharmacology Journal*, Vol. 9, no. 3 (2016), https://biomedpharmajournal.org/vol9no3/literary-review-of-parijata-nyctanthus-arbor-tristis-linn-an-herbal-medicament-with-special-reference-to-ayurveda-and-botanical-literatures/ (accessed 12 December 2024).

Kaushalendra Kumar Jha, 'Parijat: A Tree from Heaven with Confused Identity on the Gods' Earth', *Indian Forester*, Vol. 147, no. 2 (2021): 175–82, https://www.researchgate.net/publication/348907600_Parijat_A_tree_from_heaven_w

ith_confused_identity_on_the_Gods'_earth (accessed 12 December 2024).

Tapanee Hongratanaworakit, 'Stimulating Effect of Aromatherapy Massage with Jasmine Oil', *Natural Product Communications*, Vol. 5, no. 1 (2010): 157–62, https://www.researchgate.net/publication/41576755_Stimulating_Effect_of_Aromath erapy_Massage_with_Jasmine_Oil (accessed 12 December 2024).

Tsun-Cheng Kuo, 'A Study about the Inhibition Effect of Jasmine Essential Oil on the Central Nervous System', *Journal of Health Science*, Vol. 7, no. 4 (2017): 67–72, http://article.sapub.org/1 0.5923.j.health.20170704.01.html#Sec5 (accessed 30 January 2025).

Sowmyalakshmi Venkataraman et al., 'Phytochemical Constituents and Pharmacological Activities of *Nyctanthes arbor-tristis*', *Research J. Pharm. and Tech.*, Vol. 12, no. 10 (2019): 4639–43, https://rjptonline.org/HTML_Papers/Research%20 Journal%20of%20Pharmacy%20and%20Technology__ PID__2019-12-10-8.html (accessed 30 January 2025).

Chhaya S. Godse et al., 'Antiparasitic and Disease-Modifying Activity of *Nyctanthes arbor-tristis* Linn. in Malaria: An Exploratory Clinical Study', *Journal of Ayurveda and Integrative Medicine*, Vol. 7, no. 4 (2016): 238–48, https://pmc.ncbi.nlm. nih.gov/articles/PMC5192257/ (accessed 30 January 2025).

S.R. Karnik, 'Antimalarial Activity and Clinical Safety of Traditionally Used *Nyctanthes arbor-tristis* Linn.', *Indian Journal of Traditional Knowledge*, Vol. 7, no. 2 (April 2008): 330–34, https:// nopr.niscpr.res.in/bitstream/123456789/1596/1/IJTK%20 7%282%29%20330-334.pdf (accessed 30 January 2025).

Pomegranate

Edith Cowan University Research Team, 'Pomegranates Could Offer a Solution to Fatty Liver Disease', *ECU Newsroom*, 27 May 2024, https://www.ecu.edu.au/newsroom/articles/ research/pomegranates-could-offer-a-solution-to-fatty-liver-disease#:~:text=Ellegic%20acid%2C%20an%20 antioxidant%20found,caused%20by%20fatty%20liver%20 disease (accessed 12 December 2024).

Aida Zarfeshany, Sedigheh Asgary and Shaghayegh Haghjoo Javanmard, 'Potent Health Effects of Pomegranate', *Advanced Biomedical Research*, Vol. 3, no. 1 (2014): 100, https:// pmc.ncbi.nlm.nih.gov/articles/PMC4007340/ (accessed 30 January 2025).

Susanne M. Henning et al., 'Pomegranate Juice and Extract Consumption Increases the Resistance to UVB-Induced Erythema and Changes the Skin Microbiome in Healthy Women: A Randomized Controlled Trial', *Scientific Reports*, Vol. 9, 2019, https://pmc.ncbi.nlm.nih.gov/articles/ PMC6787198/ (accessed 30 January 2025).

Mohammad Reza Afroogh, 'Pomegranate and Its Properties According to the Holy Quran', *Research Journal of Food and Nutrition*, Vol. 3, no. 4 (2019): 14–17, https:// sryahwapublications.com/article/download/2637- 5583.0304003#:~:text=Pomegranates%20are%20one%20 of%20the%20paradise%20fruits%20mentioned%20in%20 the%20Holy%20Quran.&text=Quranic%20medicine%20 scholars%20believe%20that,in%20preventing%20 depression%20and%20worry. (accessed 30 January 2025).

Patricia Langley, 'Why a Pomegranate?', *British Medical Journal*, November 2000, https://pmc.ncbi.nlm.nih.gov/articles/ PMC1118911/#:~:text=Before%20its%20medicinal%20 properties%20were,life%2C%20regeneration%2C%20 and%20marriage. (accessed 30 January 2025).

Makayla Bezzant, 'Pomegranate Imagery: A Symbol of Conquest and Victory', *Studia Antiqua*, Vol. 18, no. 1 (July 2019): 9–15, https://scholarsarchive.byu.edu/cgi/viewcontent.cgi?article=1 262&context=studiaantiqua (accessed 30 January 2025).

Dina M. Ezz El-Din and Sahar Farouk Elkasrawy, 'Pomegranates of Ancient Egypt: Representations, Uses and Religious Significance' (paper presented during proceedings of the Fourth British Egyptology Congress at University of Manchester, 7–9 September 2018), https://www.researchgate.net/ publication/344460047_Pomegranates_of_ancient_Egypt_ representations_uses_and_religious_significance (accessed 30 January 2025).

Rice and Barley

Saikat Sen, Raja Chakraborty and Pratap Kalita, 'Rice – Not Just a Staple Food: A Comprehensive Review on Its Phytochemicals and Therapeutic Potential', *Trends in Food Science & Technology*, Vol. 97, March 2020: 265–85, https://www.sciencedirect.com/science/article/abs/pii/S0924224419300548 (accessed 30 January 2025).

Rathna Priya T. S. et al., 'Nutritional and Functional Properties of Coloured Rice Varieties of South India: A Review', *Journal of Ethnic Foods*, Vol. 6, October 2019, https://journalofethnicfoods.biomedcentral.com/articles/10.1186/s42779-019-0017-3 (accessed 30 January 2025).

Yawen Zeng et al., 'Preventive and Therapeutic Role of Functional Ingredients of Barley Grass for Chronic Diseases in Human Beings', *Oxidative Medicine and Cellular Longevity*, ed. Rodrigo Valenzuela, Vol. 2018, no. 1 (April 2018), https://pmc.ncbi.nlm.nih.gov/articles/PMC5904770/ (accessed 30 January 2025).

Subhash Chander Ahuja and Uma Ahuja, 'Rice in Religion and Tradition', (paper presented at 2nd International Rice Congress, New Delhi, November 2017), https://www.researchgate.net/profile/Subhash-Ahuja/publication/321334487_Rice_in_Religion_and_Tradition/links/5bf4de87a6fdcc3a8de62413/Rice-in-Religion-and-Tradition.pdf (accessed 30 January 2025).

Yang Jing Qing and Maman Lesmana, 'Hindu-Buddhist Influence on the Myths of Rice Gods in Southeast Asia and Its Role in Modern Agriculture Development', *International Journal of Research and Innovation in Social Science*, Vol. VI, no. III (March 2022): 589–97, https://rsisinternational.org/journals/ijriss/Digital-Library/volume-6-issue-3/589-597.pdf (accessed 30 January 2025).

Emiko Ohnuki-Tierney, 'Rice as Self: Japanese Identities through Time', *Education About Asia*, Vol. 9, no. 3 (2004), https://

www.asianstudies.org/publications/eaa/archives/rice-as-self-japanese-identities-through-time/ (accessed 30 January 2025).

Rati Mohan Tripura, 'The Importance of Chowak in the Rituals of the Twiprasa in Tripura: An Ethnographic Study', *International Journal for Multidisciplinary Research*, Vol. 5, no. 5 (2023), https://www.ijfmr.com/papers/2023/5/6358.pdf (accessed 30 January 2025).

Laura Matson et al., 'Transforming Research and Relationships through Collaborative Tribal-University Partnerships on Manoomin (Wild Rice)', *Environmental Science & Policy*, Vol. 115, January 2021: 108–15, https://www.sciencedirect.com/science/article/pii/S1462901120313599 (accessed 30 January 2025).

Caroline S. Weckerle et al., 'The Role of Barley among the Shuhi in the Tibetan Cultural Area of the Eastern Himalayas', *Economic Botany*, Vol. 59, no. 4 (December 2005): 386–90, https://www.researchgate.net/publication/226579303_The_Role_of_Barley_among_the_Shuhi_in_the_Tibetan_Cultural_Area_of_the_Eastern_Himalayas (accessed 30 January 2025).

A. Badr et al., 'On the Origin and Domestication History of Barley (*Hordeum vulgare*)', *Molecular Biology and Evolution*, Vol. 17, no. 4 (April 2000): 499–510, https://pubmed.ncbi.nlm.nih.gov/10742042/ (accessed 30 January 2025).

Lotus and Hibiscus

Rohit Kumar, 'A Treasure Trove of Nutrients: Lotus Root', ResearchGate, December 2022, https://www.researchgate.net/publication/373603554_A_treasure_trove_of_nutrients_Lotus_Root (accessed 12 December 2024).

Jiao-Kun Li and Shuang-Quan Huang, 'Effective Pollinators of Asian Sacred Lotus (*Nelumbo nucifera*): Contemporary Pollinators May Not Reflect the Historical Pollination Syndrome', *Annals of Botany*, Vol. 104, no. 5 (2009): 845–51, https://pmc.ncbi.nlm.nih.gov/articles/PMC2749538/ (accessed 30 January 2025).

Hang Yang et al., 'Lotus (*Nelumbo nucifera*): A Multidisciplinary Review of Its Cultural, Ecological, and Nutraceutical Significance', *Bioresources and Bioprocessing*, Vol. 11, January

2024, https://pmc.ncbi.nlm.nih.gov/articles/PMC10991372/ (accessed 30 January 2025).

Pablito M. Magdalita and Alangelico O. San Pascual, 'Hibiscus (*Hibiscus rosa-sinensis*): Importance and Classification', *Floriculture and Ornamental Plants*, ed. S.K. Datta and Y.C. Gupta, 2022: 483–522 , https://www.researchgate.net/publication/361784592_Hibiscus_Hibiscus_rosa- sinensis_Importance_and_Classification (accessed 12 December 2024).

Nguyen Chi Thanh et al., '*Hibiscus rosa-sinensis* as a Potential Hyperaccumulator in Metal Contaminated Magnesite Mine Tailings', *Chemosphere*, Vol. 339, October 2023, https://www.sciencedirect.com/science/article/abs/pii/S0045653523020052 (accessed 30 January 2025).

Paviithraa P. and Uma Mageshwari S., 'Pharmacological Benefits of *Hibiscus rosa- sinensis* Flower', *World Journal of Pharmacy and Pharmaceutical Sciences*, Vol. 9, no. 9 (2020): 662–72, https://www.researchgate.net/publication/378240034_PHARMACOLOGICAL_BEN EFITS_OF_HIBISCUS_ROSA-SINESIS_FLOWER (accessed 12 December 2024).

William E. Ward, 'The Lotus Symbol: Its Meaning in Buddhist Art and Philosophy', *Journal of Aesthetics and Art Criticism*, Vol. 11, no. 2 (December 1952): 135–46, https://www.jstor.org/stable/426039 (accessed 12 December 2024).

R.N. Mandal and R. Bar, 'The Sacred Lotus: An Incredible Wealth of Wetlands', *Resonance*, August 2013, pp. 732–37, https://www.ias.ac.in/article/fulltext/reso/018/08/0732-0737 (accessed 12 December 2024).

Sesame, Turmeric and Mustard

Anisha Mazumder, Anupma Dwivedi and Jeanetta du Plessis, 'Sinigrin and Its Therapeutic Benefits', *Molecules*, ed. Christopher W.K. Lam, Vol. 21, no. 4 (March 2016), https://pmc.ncbi.nlm.nih.gov/articles/PMC6273501/ (accessed 30 January 2025).

Kavita H. Poddar et al., 'Mustard Oil and Cardiovascular Health: Why the Controversy?', *Journal of Clinical Lipidology*, Vol. 16, no. 1 (2022): 13–22, https://www.sciencedirect.com/science/article/abs/pii/S1933287421002609 (accessed 30 January 2025).

Gitishree Das et al., 'Glucosinolates and Omega-3 Fatty Acids from Mustard Seeds: Phytochemistry and Pharmacology', *Plants*, ed. Vincenzo D'Amelia, Massimo Iorizzo and Teresa Docimo, Vol. 11, no. 17 (2022), https://pmc.ncbi.nlm.nih.gov/articles/PMC9459965/ (accessed 30 January 2025).

Magisetty Obulesu, 'Health Benefits of Turmeric: Emphasis on Anticancer Activity', *Turmeric and Curcumin for Neurodegenerative Diseases* (2021), https://www.sciencedirect.com/topics/neuroscience/turmerone#:~:text=Turmerones%20are%20the%20principal%20sesquiterpenes,enhancing%20the%20bioavailability%20of%20curcumin. (accessed 30 January 2025).

N.C. Shah, '*Sesamum indicum* (Sesame or *Til*): Seeds and Oil – An Historical and Scientific Evaluation from Indian Perspective', *Indian Journal of History of Science*, Vol. 48, no. 2 (2013): 151–74, https://cahc.jainuniversity.ac.in/assets/ijhs/Vol48_2_1_NCShah.pdf (accessed 30 January 2025).

Dorothea Bedigian, 'History and Lore of Sesame in Southwest Asia', *Economic Botany*, Vol. 58, no. 3 (2004): 329–53, https://www.jstor.org/stable/4256831?read-now=1&seq=6#page_scan_tab_contents (accessed 30 January 2025).

Shreedevi H. Huddar, E. Anupkumar and Anil Jadhav, 'Classical Review of *Haridra* (*Curcuma longa*)', *Journal of Ayurveda and Integrated Medical Sciences*, Vol. 8, no. 4 (April 2023), https://jaims.in/jaims/article/view/2409/3240 (accessed 30 January 2025).

David E. Sopher, 'Indigenous Uses of Turmeric (*Curcuma domestica*) in Asia and Oceania', *Anthropos*, Vol. 59, 1964: 93–127, https://www.jstor.org/stable/40456285?read-now=1&seq=2#page_scan_tab_contents (accessed 30 January 2025).

Aparajita and Crown Flower

Mazen A.M. Al Sulaibi, Carolin Thiemann and Thies Thiemann, 'Chemical Constituents and Uses of *Calotropis procera* and

C. gigantea – A Review (Part I – The Plants as Material and Energy Resources)', *Open Chemistry Journal*, Vol. 7, April 2020: 1–15, https://benthamopenarchives.com/abstract.php?ArticleCode=CHEM-7-1 (accessed 30 January 2025).

Prativa Biswasroy et al., 'Pharmacological Investigation of *Calotropis gigantea*: A Benevolent Herb of Nature', *Research Journal of Pharmacy and Technology*, Vol. 13, no. 1 (2020): 461–67, https://rjptonline.org/HTMLPaper.aspx?Journal=Research+Journal+of+Pharmacy+and+Technology%3bPID%3d2020-13-1-90 (accessed 30 January 2025).

Malaya K. Misra, Manoj K. Mohanty and Pradeep K. Das, 'Studies on the Method – Ethnobotany of *Calotropis gigantea* and *C. procera*', *Ancient Sciences of Life*, Vol. XIII, no. 1 and 2 (1993): 40–56, https://pmc.ncbi.nlm.nih.gov/articles/PMC3336534/pdf/ASL-13-40.pdf (accessed 30 January 2025).

Augustine Amalraj et al., 'Biological Activities of Curcuminoids, Other Biomolecules from Turmeric and Their Derivatives – A Review', *Journal of Traditional and Complementary Medicine*, Vol. 7, no. 2 (2016): 205–33, https://pmc.ncbi.nlm.nih.gov/articles/PMC5388087/#:~:text=Two%20active%20components%20of%20turmeric,specific%20for%20the%20Curcuma%20genus. (accessed 30 January 2025).

Pulok K. Mukherjee et al., 'The Ayurvedic Medicine *Clitoria ternatea*–from Traditional Use to Scientific Assessment', *Journal of Ethnopharmacology*, Vol. 120, no. 3 (December 2008): 291–301, https://pubmed.ncbi.nlm.nih.gov/18926895/#:~:text=Clitoria%20ternatea%20L.,anticonvulsant%2C%20tranquilizing%20and%20sedative%20agent. (accessed 30 January 2025).

Deepika Sahu et al., 'Phytochemicals and Medicinal Uses of *Clitoria ternatea*', *International Journal of Plant & Soil Science*, Vol. 35, no. 18 (2023): 942–51, https://journalijpss.com/index.php/IJPSS/article/view/3405 (accessed 30 January 2025).

Babita Patial et al., 'A Review on Biological Activities of Indian Traditional Medicinal Plant: *Calotropis gigantea*', *Journal of Biomedical and Allied Research*, Vol. 4, no. 2 (2022), https://maplespub.com/article/a-review-on-biological-activities-of-indian-traditional-medicinal-plant-calotropis-gigantea (accessed 30 January 2025).

PART III

Rudraksha and Tulsi

Anisha S. Ashraf, 'Rudraksha: Therapeutic Approach in Ayurveda', *Paripex – Indian Journal of Research*, Vol. 8, no. 6 (June 2019): 34–37, https://www.worldwidejournals.com/paripex/recent_issues_pdf/2019/June/June_2019_1559719490_1701447.pdf (accessed 31 January 2025).

Shailja Choudhary and Hemlata Kaurav, '*Elaeocarpus ganitrus* (Rudraksha): A Drug with Spiritual and Medicinal Properties', *International Journal of Pharmacy and Biological Sciences*, Vol. 11, no. 3 (2021): 242–53, https://www.ijpbs.com/ijpbsadmin/upload/ijpbs_61b5b05c9972f.pdf (accessed 31 January 2025).

Swati Hardainiyan, Bankim Chandra Nandy and Krishan Kumar, '*Elaeocarpus ganitrus* (Rudraksha): A Reservoir Plant with Their Pharmacological Effects', *International Journal of Pharmaceutical Sciences Review and Research*, Vol. 34, no. 1 (2015): 55–64, https://globalresearchonline.net/journalcontents/v34-1/10.pdf (accessed 31 January 2025).

Shiva Sharma, Durg V. Rai and Manisha Rastogi, 'Magnetic Characteristics of Different Mukhi Rudraksha Beads: A Comparative Analysis', *International Journal of Scientific and Technology Research*, Vol. 8, no. 11 (2019): 3329–33, https://www.ijstr.org/final-print/nov2019/Magnetic-Characteristics-Of-Different-Mukhi-Rudraksha-Beads-A-Comparative-Analysis.pdf (accessed 12 December 2024).

Shiva Sharma et al., 'Electrical Behavior of Plant Based Material', *Materials Today: Proceedings*, Vol. 79, 2023: 349–54, https://www.sciencedirect.com/science/article/abs/pii/S2214785322074053 (accessed 31 January 2025).

Héctor Calderón Bravo et al., 'Basil Seeds as a Novel Food, Source of Nutrients and Functional Ingredients with Beneficial Properties:

A Review', *Foods*, vol. 10, no. 7 (2021), https://pmc.ncbi.nlm. nih.gov/articles/PMC8303141/ (accessed 31 January 2025).

Subhashish Tripathy, Amit Mishra and Arun Kumar Mishra, 'The Unexplained Negative Electromagnetic Radiation and Its Reduction Effect on Human by Electromagnetic Seed Rudraksha', *Journal of Drug Delivery & Therapeutics*, Vol. 11, no. 3 (2021): 48–52, https://jddtonline.info/index.php/jddt/article/view/4881 (accessed 12 December 2024).

T.V.R.S. Sharma et al., 'Gardening of *Elaeocarpus* (Rudraksha) for Conservation and Tourist Interest in Andaman and Nicobar Islands', *Journal of the Andaman Science Association*, Vol. 20, no. 2 (2015): 172–77, https://krishi.icar.gov.in/jspui/bitstream/123456789/19763/1/eLAEOCARPUS%20 GARDENING.pdf (accessed 31 January 2025).

Babita Kumari, Apurva Srivastava and Santosh Kumar Tiwari, '*Elaeocarpus* spp.: A Threatened Power Generating Plant, Its Geographical Distribution, Propagation through *In Vivo* Condition and Its Medicinal Aspects', *International Journal of Fauna and Biological Studies*, Vol. 5, no. 2 (2018): 27–31, https://www.faunajournal.com/archives/2018/vol5issue2/ PartA/5-2-3-945.pdf (accessed 31 January 2025).

Negar Jamshidi and Marc M. Cohen, 'The Clinical Efficacy and Safety of Tulsi in Humans: A Systematic Review of the Literature', *Evidence-Based Complementary and Alternative Medicine*, ed. Daniela Rigano, Vol. 2017, no. 1 (2017), https:// pmc.ncbi.nlm.nih.gov/articles/PMC5376420/ (accessed 31 January 2025).

Durva Grass and Arjun

Tarun Virmani et al., 'Hidden Potential of Doob Grass: An Indian Traditional Drug', *Research in Pharmacy and Health Sciences*, Vol. 4, no. 3 (2018): 478–82, https://www.researchgate.net/publication/328225354_Hidden_Potential_of_Doob_Gr ass-An_Indian_Traditional_Drug (accessed 12 December 2024).

V. Harini and Sonu Joseph, 'Mythology and Medicine: A Comparative Study of Native American's Sweet Grass and Indian's *Durva*

REFERENCES

Grass', *Journal of Natural Remedies*, Vol. 23, no. 4 (2023), https://www.researchgate.net/publication/375631290_Mythology_and_Medicine_A_ Comparative_Study_of_Native_American's_Sweet_Grass_and_Indian's_Durva_Grass (accessed 12 December 2024).

Satya Prakash Chaudhary et al., 'An Ayurvedic Review of Arjuna from Samhita', *International Journal of Research in Ayurveda and Pharmacy*, Vol. 8, 2017, https://www.researchgate.net/publication/317689337_AN_AYURVEDIC_REVIEW_ OF_ARJUNA_FROM_SAMHITA (accessed 12 December 2024).

Sahil Gupta, 'Durva (*Cynodon dactylon*): Uses and Benefits', November 2023, https://www.iafaforallergy.com/herbs-a-to-z/durva- cynodondactylon/ (accessed 12 December 2024).

'Durva (Grass)', https://ishanayurved.com/medicinal-plants/durva-grass/ (accessed 12 December 2024).

Sheetal Yadav et al., '*Terminalia arjuna* (Arjun Tree): A Sacred Plant with High Medicinal and Therapeutic Potential', *Research Journal of Pharmacy and Technology*, Vol. 15, no. 12 (2022), https://rjptonline.org/AbstractView.aspx?PID=2022-15-12-83#:~:text=arjuna%20has%20antimutagenic%2C%20cardioprotective%2C%20hyper,%2C%20antifungal%2C%20and%20antibacterial%20properties. (accessed 12 December 2024).

Vikas Kumar et al., 'Therapeutic Potential and Industrial Applications of *Terminalia arjuna* Bark', *Journal of Ethnopharmacology*, Vol. 310, June 2023, https://pubmed.ncbi.nlm.nih.gov/36933876/ (accessed 31 January 2025).

Huaguo Liang et al., 'Methyl Gallate: Review of Pharmacological Activity', *Pharmacological Research*, Vol. 194, August 2023, https://www.sciencedirect.com/science/article/pii/S1043661823002050 (accessed 31 January 2025).

Savita S. Angadi and Sumitra T. Gowda, 'Management of *Vyanga* (Facial Melanosis) with *Arjuna Twak Lepa* and *Panchanimba Churna*', *Ayu (An International Quarterly Journal of Research in Ayurveda)*, Vol. 35, no. 1 (2014): 50–53, https://pmc.ncbi.nlm.nih.gov/articles/PMC4213969/ (accessed 31 January 2025).

Shami and Bael

Prabhavathi Dharani, B.R. Lalitha and K. Kala, 'Shami (*Prosopis cineraria* (L) Druce): A Medicinal Benison', *Journal of Ayurveda and Integrated Medical Sciences*, Vol. 5, no. 5 (2020): 441–48, https://jaims.in/jaims/article/view/1081 (accessed 12 December 2024).

S. Monika, M. Thirumal and P.R. Kumar, 'Phytochemical and Biological Review of *Aegle marmelos* Linn', *Future Science OA*, Vol. 9, no. 3 (2023), https://pmc.ncbi.nlm.nih.gov/articles/PMC10072075/ (accessed 31 January 2025).

Prabodh Chander Sharma et al., 'A Review on Bael Tree', *Natural Product Radiance*, Vol. 6, no. 2 (2007): 171–78, https://www.doc-developpement-durable.org/file/Culture/Arbres-Fruitiers/FICHES_ARBRES/Bael/A%20review%20on%20Bael%20tree.pdf (accessed 31 January 2025).

V.N. Ariharan and P. Nagendra Prasad, '"*Mahavilva*" A Sacred Tree with Immense Medicinal Secrets: A Mini Review', *Rasāyan Journal of Chemistry*, Vol. 6, no. 4 (2013): 342–52, https://www.researchgate.net/publication/260150552_'Mahavilva'_a_sacred_tree_with_immense_medicinal_secrets_A_mini_review (accessed 31 January 2025).

Shailja Choudhary, Gitika Chaudhary and Hemlata Kaurav, '*Aegle Marmelos* (Bael Patra): An Ayurvedic Plant with Ethnomedicinal Value', *International Journal of Research in Ayurveda and Pharmacy*, Vol. 12, no. 3 (2021): 147–49, https://www.researchgate.net/publication/353022468_AEGLE_MARMELOS_BAEL_PATRA_AN_AYURVEDIC_PLANT_WITH_ETHNOMEDICINAL_VALUE (accessed 31 January 2025).

Jamun and Jackfruit

Manoj Kumar et al., 'Jamun (*Syzygium cumini* (L.) Skeels) Seed Bioactives and Its Biological Activities: A Review', *Food Bioscience*, Vol. 50, December 2022, https://www.sciencedirect.com/science/article/abs/pii/S2212429222005697#:~:text=J

amun%20(Syzygium%20cumini%20Skeels)%20is,them%20 valuable%20components%20of%20nutraceuticals (accessed 12 December 2024).

R.A.S.N. Ranasinghe, S.D.T. Maduwanthi and R.A.U.J. Marapana, 'Nutritional and Health Benefits of Jackfruit (*Artocarpus heterophyllus* Lam.): A Review', *International Journal of Food Science*, ed. Amy Simonne, Vol. 2019, no. 1 (2019), https:// pmc.ncbi.nlm.nih.gov/articles/PMC6339770/ (accessed 31 January 2025).

Kathleen Weintraub, Camila Rodrigues and Katia Tabai, 'Perspectives on Sustainable Management of Jackfruit Trees for Food Consumption in Rio de Janeiro, Brazil', *Environmental Science Proceedings*, Vol. 15, no. 1 (2022), https://www.mdpi. com/2673-4931/15/1/8 (accessed 31 January 2025).

Apurva Rai et al., 'The Importance of *Butea monosperma* for the Restoration of Degraded Lands', *Ecological Engineering*, Vol. 97, December 2016: 619–23, https://www.sciencedirect.com/ science/article/abs/pii/S0925857416305602 (accessed 31 January 2025).

Palash and Kachnar

Pooja Singh et al., 'A Review on Bramhavriksha: Palash (*Butea Monosperma*)', World Journal of Pharmaceutical and Life Sciences, Vol. 9, no. 4 (2023): 100–09, https://www.wjpls. org/download/article/91032023/1680586462.pdf (accessed 31 January 2025).

Hirdayesh Anuragi et al., *Palash (Butea monosperma): A Monograph* (Jhansi: ICAR-CAFRI, 2023), pp. 1–128, https://www. researchgate.net/publication/376413855_Palash_Butea_ monosperma_A_Monograph (accessed 31 January 2025).

Isha Kumari, Hemlata Kaurav and Gitika Choudhary, 'Bauhinia Variegate (Kanchnara): An Ornamental Plant with Significant Value in Ayurvedic and Folk Medicinal System', *Himalayan Journal of Health Sciences*, Vol. 6, no. 2 (2021), https://www.researchgate.net/publication/353264218_ Bauhinia_variegata_Kanchnara_An_ornamental_Plant_ with_significant_value_in_Ayurvedic_and_Folk_Medicinal_system (accessed 12 December 2024).

Shikha Tiwari and Vaibhav Acharya, 'Sacred Trees of Raipur City', *International Journal of Life Sciences Research*, Vol. 7, no. 2 (2019): 119 –128, https://www.researchpublish.com/upload/book/SACRED%20TREES%20OF%20RAIPUR%20CITY-7392.pdf (accessed 31 January 2025).

Apurva Rai et al., '*Butea monosperma*: A Leguminous Species for Sustainable Forestry Programmes', *Environment, Development and Sustainability*, Vol. 23, no. 1 (2021): 8492–505, https://www.researchgate.net/publication/345306617_Butea_monosperma_a_leguminous_species_for_sustainable_forestry_programmes (accessed 31 January 2025).

Muhammad Yasir Naeem and Senay Ugur, 'Nutritional and Health Consequences of Bauhinia variegata', *Turkish Journal of Agriculture – Food Science and Technology*, Vol. 7, no. 3 (2019): 27–30, https://www.researchgate.net/publication/338402465_Nutritional_and_Health_Consequences_of_Bauhinia_variegata (accessed 31 January 2025).

R. Verma et al., 'Effect of Maturity on the Physico-Chemical and Nutritional Characteristics of *Kachnar* (*Bauhinia variegata* Linn.) Green Buds and Flowers', *Indian Journal of Natural Products and Resources*, Vol. 3, no. 2 (2012): 242–45, https://nopr.niscpr.res.in/bitstream/123456789/14407/1/IJNPR%203(2)%20242-245.pdf (accessed 31 January 2025).

Mahua and Sal

D. Thangamani et al., 'Spiritually Significant Natural Resource of *Madhuca longifolia* (J. Koenig ex L.) J.F. Macbr. Conservation and Its Value Added Products Management', *Pharma Innovation Journal*, Vol. 11, no. 8 (2022): 792–96, https://www.researchgate.net/publication/363923544_Spiritually_significant_natural_resource_of_Madhuca_longifolia_J_Koenig_ex_L_JF_Macbr_conservation_and_its_value_added_products_management (accessed 12 December 2024).

Ramdev Jurri and Farhad Mollick, 'Ethnographical Study of Religious Significance of Mahua in Tribal Community', *International Journal of Social Science and Management Studies*, Vol. 7, no. 8 (2021), https://www.researchgate.net/publication/369184370_Ethnographical_Study_of_Religious_Significance_of_Mahua_in_Tribal_Community (accessed 12 December 2024).

Gautam Kumar Das, 'Mahua Tree and Its Products', *Indian Science Cruiser*, Vol. 36, no. 4 (July 2022): 11–12, https://www.researchgate.net/publication/366157311_Mahua_Tree_and_Its_Products (accessed 12 December 2024).

Sheetal et al., 'A Review on Importance of Sal Tree (*Shorea robusta*) as an Interminable Wood', *Asian Journal of Microbiology, Biotechnology and Environmental Sciences*, Vol. 26, no. 1 (2024): 153–56, https://www.researchgate.net/publication/380147403_A_REVIEW_ON_IMPORTANCE_OF_SAL_TREE_SHOREA_ROBUSTA_AS_AN_INTERMINABLE_WOOD (accessed 12 December 2024).

Hari Shankar Lal, Sanjay Singh and Mishra P.K., 'Trees in Indian Mythology', *Discovery*, Vol. 12, no. 29 (2014): 16–23, https://www.discoveryjournals.org/discovery/current_issue/v11-13/n25-34/A8.pdf (accessed 31 January 2025).

Areej Fatma et al., 'Evaluation of Antibacterial Activity of Madhuca longifolia (Mahua) Stem Extract Against Streptococcus mutans: An In Vitro Study', *Cureus*, ed. Alexander Muacevic and John R. Adler, Vol. 16, no. 1 (2024), https://pmc.ncbi.nlm.nih.gov/articles/PMC10860734/ (accessed 31 January 2025).

Dave Jaydeep Pinakin et al., 'Mahua: A Boon for Pharmacy and Food Industry', *Current Research in Nutrition and Food Science*, Vol. 6, no. 2 (2018), https://www.foodandnutritionjournal.org/volume6number2/mahua-a-boon-for-pharmacy-and-food-industry/ (accessed 31 January 2025).

Vishal Johar and Rupender Kumar, 'Mahua: A Versatile Indian Tree Species', *Journal of Pharmacognosy and Phytochemistry*, Vol. 9, no. 6 (2020): 1926–31, https://www.researchgate.net/publication/347947468_Mahua_A_versatile_Indian_tree_species (accessed 12 December 2024).

Smruti Ranjan Das, Rajkumari Supriya Devi and Sanjeet Kumar, 'Ecological, Cultural and Medicinal Values of Sal (*Shorea robusta*): A Multifaceted Native Tree of India', *Ethnopharmacology*, Vol. I, 2024: 8–17, https://www.researchgate.net/publication/379759074_ECOLOGICAL_CULTURAL_ AND_MEDICINAL_VALUES_OF_SAL_Shorea_robusta_A_MULTIFACETED_N ATIVE_TREE_OF_INDIA (accessed 12 December 2024).

Neem and Amla

Alim Nisa, Sajawal Ashraf and Fatima Sajjad, *Neem Tree: A Sacred Gift of Nature* (Noor Publishing, 2021), https://www.researchgate.net/publication/357528444_Neem_tree_A_Sacred_Gift_of_Nature#:~:text=Moreover%2C%20Neem%20tree%20is%20considered,application%2	0in%20agriculture%20or%20Agroforestry (accessed 12 December 2024).

Venugopalan Santhosh Kumar and Visweswaran Navaratnam, 'Neem (*Azadirachta indica*): Prehistory to Contemporary Medicinal Uses to Humankind', *Asian Pacific Journal of Tropical Biomedicine*, Vol. 3, no. 7 (2013): 505–14, https://pmc.ncbi.nlm.nih.gov/articles/PMC3695574/ (accessed 31 January 2025).

'About Neem: History of Usage', Neem Foundation, https://neemfoundation.org/about-neem/history-of-usage/ (accessed 31 January 2025).

Ekta Singh et al., 'Phytochemistry, Traditional Uses and Cancer Chemopreventive Activity of Amla (*Phyllanthus emblica*): The Sustainer', *Journal of Applied Pharmaceutical Science*, Vol. 2, no. 1 (2011): 176–83, https://japsonline.com/admin/php/uploads/365_pdf.pdf (accessed 12 December 2024).

Gowthami S. and Thirumoorthy R., 'Studies on Development of Amla and Its Products: A Review', *International Journal of Advances in Engineering and Management*, Vol. 3, no. 5 (May 2021): 992–96, https://ijaem.net/issue_dcp/Studieson%20Development%20of%20Amla%20and%20Its%20Products%20A%20Review.pdf (accessed 12 December 2024).

REFERENCES

Snehal S. Pawar et al., 'A Pharmacological Review on Amla (*emblica*)', *International Journal of Creative Research Thoughts*, Vol. 9, no. 2 (2021): 3482–88, https://ijcrt.org/papers/IJCRT2102417.pdf (accessed 31 January 2025).

Jose Francisco Islas et al., 'An Overview of Neem (*Azadirachta indica*) and Its Potential Impact on Health', *Journal of Functional Foods*, Vol. 74, November 2020, https://www.sciencedirect.com/science/article/pii/S1756464620303959 (accessed 31 January 2025).

S. Gajalakshmi and S.A. Abbasi, 'Neem Leaves as a Source of Fertilizer-cum-Pesticide Vermicompost', *Bioresource Technology*, Vol. 92, no. 3 (May 2004): 291–96, https://www.sciencedirect.com/science/article/abs/pii/S0960852403002438 (accessed 31 January 2025).

Rajendra Prasad and Samendra Prasad, 'Neem and the Environment', *International Journal of Plant and Environment*, Vol. 4, no. 1 (January 2018): 1–9, https://www.researchgate.net/publication/338967716_Neem_and_the_Environment (accessed 31 January 2025).

Maryam Gul et al., 'Functional and Nutraceutical Significance of Amla (*Phyllanthus emblica* L.): A Review', *Antioxidants*, Vol. 11, no. 5 (April 2022), https://pmc.ncbi.nlm.nih.gov/articles/PMC9137578/ (accessed 31 January 2025).

Abhishek Maitry et al., 'Ecological and Economic Potential of Amla (*Phyllanthus emblica* L.): A Horticulture Crop for Degraded Land Restoration, Food Security and Sustainable Livelihood in Chhattisgarh, India', *Chhattisgarh Journal of Science and Technology*, Vol. 19, no. 3 (2022): 123–27, https://www.researchgate.net/publication/372449968_Ecological_and_Economic_Potential_of_Amla_Phyllanthus_emblica_L_A_Horticulture_Crop_for_Degraded_Land_Restoration_Food_Security_and_Sustainable_Livelihood_in_Chhattisgarh_India (accessed 31 January 2025).

Kadamba and Ashoka

Arti Pandey and Pradeep Singh Negi, 'Traditional Uses, Phytochemistry and Pharmacological Properties of *Neo`lamarckia cadamba*: A Review', *Journal of Ethnopharmacology*, Vol. 181, April 2016: 118–35, https://www.sciencedirect.com/science/article/abs/pii/S0378874116300368 (accessed 31 January 2025).

Ranjan Kumar Singh et al., 'Botanical Description, Phytochemistry, Traditional Uses, and Pharmacology of *Anthocephalus cadamba*: An Updated Review', *World Journal of Biology Pharmacy and Health Sciences*, Vol. 12, no. 3 (2022): 132–45, https://www.researchgate.net/publication/366352714_Botanical_description_phytoch emistry_traditional_uses_and_pharmacology_of_Anthocephalus_cadamba_An_updat ed_review (accessed 12 December 2024).

Hari Shankar Lal, Sanjay Singh and Mishra P.K., 'Trees in Indian Mythology', *Discovery*, Vol. 12, no. 29 (2014): 16–23, https://www.discoveryjournals.org/discovery/current_issue/v11-13/n25-34/A8.pdf (accessed 31 January 2025).

Sumanta Mondal et al., '"Haripriya" God's Favorite: *Anthocephalus cadamba* (Roxb.) Miq. – At a Glance', *Pharmacognosy Research*, Vol. 12, no. 1 (2020): 1–16, https://www.phcogres.com/sites/default/files/PharmacognRes-12-1-1.pdf (accessed 12 December 2024).

Satish A. Bhalerao, '*Saraca asoca* (Roxb.), De. Wild: An Overview', *Annals of Plant Sciences*, Vol. 3, no. 7 (2014): 770–75, https://www.researchgate.net/publication/304173094_Saraca_asoca_Roxb_De_Wild_An_overview (accessed 12 December 2024).

Vidit Parkar et al., '*Polyalthia longifolia* (False Ashoka) is an Ideal Choice for Better Air Quality at Kerbside Locations' (paper presented at EGU General Assembly, May 2020), https://www.researchgate.net/publication/344247492_Polyalthia_longifolia_False_As hoka_is_an_ideal_choice_for_better_air_quality_at_kerbside_locations (accessed 12 December 2024).

Arti Pandey et al., 'Proximate and Mineral Composition of Kadamba (*Neolamarckia cadamba*) Fruit and Its Use in the Development of Nutraceutical Enriched Beverage', *Journal of Food Science and Technology*, Vol. 55, 2018: 4330–36, https://pmc.ncbi.nlm.nih.gov/articles/PMC6133846/ (accessed 31 January 2025).

REFERENCES

Tamarind

Md. Salim Azad, 'Tamarindo – *Tamarindus indica*', *Exotic Fruits*, 2018: 403–12, https://www.sciencedirect.com/science/article/abs/pii/B9780128031384000551 (accessed 31 January 2025).

Mohan Maruga Raja et al., 'A Scientific Evidence-Based Review of Tamarind Usage in Indian Folklore Medicine', *Journal of Natural Remedies*, Vol. 22, no. 3 (July 2022): 347–62, https://www.researchgate.net/publication/364261720_A_Scientific_Evidence-based_Review_of_Tamarind_usage_in_Indian_Folklore_Medicine (accessed 31 January 2025).

Reinout M. Havinga et al., '*Tamarindus indica* L. (Fabaceae): Patters of Use in Traditional African Medicine', *Journal of Ethnopharmacology*, Vol. 127, no. 3 (February 2010): 573–88, https://www.sciencedirect.com/science/article/abs/pii/S0378874109007351 (accessed 31 January 2025).

Hailay Girmay et al., 'Use and Management of Tamarind (*Tamarindus indica* L., Fabaceae) Local Morphotypes by Communities in Tigray, Northern Ethiopia', *Forests, Trees and Livelihoods*, Vol. 29, no. 2 (2020): 81–98, https://www.researchgate.net/publication/339812932_Use_and_management_of_tamarind_Tamarindus_indica_L_Fabaceae_local_morphotypes_by_communities_in_Tigray_Northern_Ethiopia (accessed 31 January 2025).

Pinar Kuru, '*Tamarindus indica* and Its Health-Related Effects', *Asian Pacific Journal of Tropical Biomedicine*, Vol. 4, no. 9 (September 2014): 676–81, https://www.sciencedirect.com/science/article/pii/S2221169115300885 (accessed 31 January 2025).

F.A. Chimsah, G. Nyarko and A.H. Abubakari, 'A Review of Explored Uses and Study of Nutritional Potential of Tamarind (*Tamarindus indica* L.) in Northern Ghana', *African Journal of Food Science*, Vol. 14, no. 9 (October 2020): 285–94, https://academicjournals.org/journal/AJFS/article-full-text-pdf/DFE5EFE64946 (accessed 31 January 2025).

Vikram Balaji et al., 'Tamarind Cultivation, Value-Added Products and their Health Benefits: A Review', *International Journal of*

Plant and Soil Science, Vol. 35, no. 21 (2023): 903–11, https://www.researchgate.net/publication/375413344_Tamarind_Cultivation_Value-Added_Products_and_Their_Health_Benefits_A_Review (accessed 31 January 2025).

Chinar and Deodar

Rajesh K Manhas, 'The Dwindling Glory of Chinar', *Current Science*, Vol. 104, no. 11 (June 2013): 1466–67, https://www.researchgate.net/publication/293653202_The_dwindling_glory_of_china r (accessed 12 December 2024).

Ashiq Hussain, 'Preliminary Census of Chinar Trees in J&K: One-Third of J&K's State Tree Chinar Diseased or Damaged; May Be Lost in 10 Years', *Hindustan Times*, 6 July 2023, https://www.hindustantimes.com/cities/chandigarh-news/preliminary-census-reveals-18-000-diseased-chinar-trees-in-jammu-and-kashmir-experts-express-concern-101688665363863.html (accessed 12 December 2024).

Manish Grover, 'An Overview on the Ornamental Coniferous Tree *Cedrus deodara* (Roxburgh) G. Don (Himalayan Cedar)', *Journal of Ayurveda and Integrated Medical Sciences*, Vol. 6, no. 4 (2021): 291–302, https://jaims.in/jaims/article/view/1401 (accessed 31 January 2025).

Nirmal Kumar E. et al., 'Experimental Evaluation of Hypnotic and Antidepressant Effect of Pine Needles of *Cedrus deodara*', *Journal of Ayurveda and Integrative Medicine*, Vol. 14, no. 2 (2023), https://www.sciencedirect.com/science/article/pii/S0975947623000232 (accessed 31 January 2025).

Harsh Pathak et al., '*Cedrus deodara* (Roxb.): A Review on the Recent Update on its Pharmacological and Phytochemical Profile', *Royal Pharmaceutical Society Pharmacy and Pharmacology Reports*, Vol. 2, no. 3 (2023), https://academic.oup.com/rpsppr/article/2/3/rqad026/7234907# (accessed 31 January 2025).

Mohd. Afsahul Kalam et al., 'Deodar (*Cedrus deodara* (Roxb.) Loud.): Therapeutic Uses and Pharmacological Studies – A Review', *Indian Journal of Unani Medicine*, Vol. 16, no. 1 (2023):

REFERENCES

8–16, https://www.researchgate.net/publication/371691249_ DEODAR_CEDRUS_DEODARA_ROXB_LOUD_ THERAPEUTIC_USES_AND_PHARMACOLOGICAL_ STUDIES-A_REVIEW (accessed 31 January 2025).

Banyan and Peepal

Rutuja R. Sonawane, Utkarsha Shivsharan and Shruti A. Mehta, 'Ficus Religiosa (*Peepal*): A Phytochemical and Pharmacological Review', *International Journal of Pharmaceutical and Chemical Sciences*, Vol. 4, no. 3 (2015): 360–70, https://www. researchgate.net/publication/376047496_Ficus_Religiosa_ Peepal_A_Phy tochemical_and_Pharmacological_Review (accessed 12 December 2024).

Maheshkumar N. Chaudhari and Mrudula M. Chaudhari, 'Banyan Tree (Vad) – An Immortal Tree', *International Journal of Medicinal Plants and Natural Products*, Vol. 9, no. 4 (2023): 1–4, https://www.arcjournals.org/pdfs/ijmpnp/v9-i4/1.pdf (accessed 31 January 2025).

Kyu Hwan Shim, Niti Sharma and Seong Soo A. An, 'Mechanistic Insights into the Neuroprotective Potential of Sacred *Ficus* Trees', *Nutrients*, Vol. 14, no. 22 (2022), https://www.mdpi. com/2072-6643/14/22/4731 (accessed 31 January 2025).

Erum F.H. Kazi and Satish Kulkarni, 'APTI (Air Pollution Tolerance Index) of Trees in Lohagaon Area in Pune City in Different Seasons', *EPRA International Journal of Economic and Business Review*, Vol. 8, no. 12 (December 2020): 44–49, https://www.researchgate.net/publication/348253471_ APTI_AIR_POLLUTION_TOLERANCE_INDEX_OF_ TREES_IN_LOHAGAON_AREA_IN_PUNE_CITY_IN_ DIFFERENT_SEASONS (accessed 31 January 2025).

Rushikesh Ravindra Tahakik et al., 'Evaluation of Oxygen Molecule in *Ficus religiosa* by Spectrophotometer', *International Journal of Research*, Vol. 4, no. 3 (2017): 806–11, https://www. researchgate.net/publication/352814120_Evaluation_of_ Oxygen_Amount_in_ficus_religiosa (accessed 31 January 2025).

Pooja Agrahari et al., 'Ficus religiosa Tree Leaves as Bioindicators of Heavy Metals in Gorakhpur City, Uttar Pradesh, India', Pharmacognosy Journal, Vol. 10, no. 3 (2018): 416–20, https://www.phcogj.com/article/600 (accessed 31 January 2025).

Kamini Kumari et al., 'A Review on Ficus religiosa Moraceae: Distribution, Traditional Uses and Pharmacological Properties', Journal of Biomedical and Pharmaceutical Research, Vol. 11, no. 5 (2022): 45–54, https://www.researchgate.net/publication/364256273_A_Review_on_Ficus_Religiosa_Moraceae_Distribution_Traditional_Uses_and_Pharmacological_Properties (accessed 12 December 2024).

Abdalsalam Kmail et al., 'Banyan Tree – The Sacred Medicinal Tree with Potential Health and Pharmacological Benefits', International Journal of Chemical and Biochemical Sciences, Vol. 13, 2018: 52–57, https://www.researchgate.net/publication/343040482_Banyan_tree-the_sacred_medicinal_tree_with_potential_health_and_pharmacological_benefits (accessed 12 December 2024).

Princy Rana and Sheetal Chopra, 'Aerial Roots of Banyan Tree: A Promising Sustainable Source for Extraction of Fibres' (paper presented at Sangoshthi–2021, International Conference on Sustainability in Crafts and Design, IICD, Jaipur, April 2022), https://www.researchgate.net/publication/362430058_AERIAL_ROOTS_OF_BANYAN_TREE_A_PROMISING_SUSTAINABLE_SOURCE_FOR_EXTRACTION_OF_FIBRES (accessed 12 December 2024).

'Genomic Study Reveals Evolutionary Secrets of Banyan Tree', School of Integrative Biology, 8 October 2020, https://sib.illinois.edu/news/2020-10-08t000000/genomic-study-reveals-evolutionary-secrets-banyan-tree (accessed 31 January 2025).

Ritika and Nutan, 'Development of Value-Added Products from Banyan Tree (Ficus benghalensis) Fruit Powder', International Journal of Basic and Applied Sciences, Vol. 11, no. 4 (2022): 141–48, https://www.researchgate.net/publication/374700231_Development_of_Value_Added_Products_from_Banyan_ tree_Ficus_benghalensis_Fruit_Powder (accessed 12 December 2024).

Rakesh N. Chaudhari et al., 'Pharmacognostic, Phytochemical, Pharmacological Potential on Banyan Tree (*Ficus bengalensis* L.)', *International Journal of Pharmacy and Pharmaceutical Research*, Vol. 25, no. 1 (August 2022): 230–51, https://ijppr.humanjournals.com/wp-content/uploads/2022/09/18.Rakesh.N.Chaudhari-Yash.M.Mulani-Priyanka.V.-More-Abhishek.N.Nikumbh-Ansari-Imtiyaz-Ahmed-Tufail-Ahemad.pdf (accessed 31 January 2025).

Scan QR code to access the
Penguin Random House India website